The Complete Guide to Weight Loss Surgery: Your questions finally answered

Lisa Kaouk MPH, RD

Monica Bashaw MScA, RD

The Complete Guide to Weight Loss Surgery: Your questions finally answered
Written by registered dietitians: Lisa Kaouk MPH, RD & Monica Bashaw MScA, RD
Editor: Caitlin Marceau

ISBN: 1977881696
ISBN-13: 978-1977881694

Notice of Rights

For more information regarding reprints and excerpts, contact:
bariatricsurgerynutrition@gmail.com

Notice of Liability

The contents of this book are based on the experiences and opinions of the authors.
This book is intended to provide general food and nutrition information to WLS
patients. This book is not a substitute for medical advice. This book should not be
used to diagnose nor treat any medical conditions. For tailored advice and to
understand if this book is appropriate for you given your health profile, please consult
your WLS team. Consult your WLS team regularly for follow up and for any
signs/symptoms that concern you. The authors are not liable for any negative
consequences caused by following the advice in this book.

Disclaimer

Throughout this book we have chosen to use only the term 'Weight Loss Surgery'
(WLS) instead of 'Bariatric Surgery' as WLS is the more commonly used term. We
acknowledge that these terms can be used interchangeably.

Feedback

If you notice any errors in this book or have suggestions, please let us know!
Email us at bariatricsurgerynutrition@gmail.com

Acknowledgements

A big thank you to all of our volunteer editors! Your feedback was invaluable.

Dedication

This book is dedicated to all of our fabulous weight loss surgery (WLS) patients past, present and future. We admire your bravery and life-long commitment in choosing WLS to improve your health. Thank you for sharing your struggles, your tips, your doubts, your fears and your successes with us over the years. Your stories were the inspiration for this book.

- Lisa & Monica

TABLE OF CONTENTS

Chapter 3: Hunger & Appetite

Chapter 4: Water

Chapter 5: Protein

Chapter 6: Delaying Fluids

Chapter 7: Dumping Syndrome

Chapter 8: Hair Loss

Chapter 9: Alcohol

Chapter 10: Caffeine

Chapter 11: Calories & Carbs

Chapter 12: Portions & Structure

Chapter 13: Eating Out

Introduction

Hello reader!

The fact that you have this book in your hands means that you understand how big a deal weight loss surgery is. And trust us, it *is* a big deal. There's so much to know!

Why did we write this book?

A little over a year ago, we sat down and made a list of the most common questions we (as weight loss surgery dietitians) get asked every day in our clinics. Our goal for this book was to create a comprehensive FAQ style guidebook to answer all of the big questions you guys have. We wanted to create a handbook to answer the most common "Why is this important?" and the 'What do I do now?" type of questions. We had no idea that we would end up with 18 chapters so quickly!

You'll notice that most of the questions are related to food, beverages and nutrition (i.e. basically what you would expect from two dietitians!), but we have also done our best to cover the most common tolerance issues that patients run in to (e.g. nausea, vomiting, heartburn, constipation and diarrhea), along with information on 'normal' weight loss, vitamins, and emotional changes with surgery, plus tons of tips to help you stay on track.

Who is this book for?

We feel this book is relevant to ALL stages of the weight loss surgery journey. Whether you are preparing for surgery (good luck!), have recently had surgery (congrats!), are years after surgery (you can do this!), or are supporting someone through their surgery (you're awesome!), there is a TON of information for you in this book. Although a lot of the material *does* focus on issues that come up in the first 3-6 months after surgery, it still definitely provides a solid summary of the basics for those of you who are looking to refresh your habits.

How should you read this book?

Depending on where you are in your weight loss surgery journey, some sections of this book may not be relevant. For this reason, we recommend using the Table of Contents to navigate your way through the chapters. While reading, we encourage you to fold down page corners, underline relevant info, highlight tips that resonate with you, etc. to get the most out of this book.

We sincerely wish you the best of luck in your WLS journey!

Lisa Kaouk, MPH, RD & Monica Bashaw, MScA, RD
Co-founders of Bariatric Surgery Nutrition
www.bariatricsurgerynutrition.com

CHAPTER 1:

Weight Loss

Body weight vocabulary, some useful definitions

best **EXCESS** BMI

NORMAL WEIGHT

ideal *expected*

It can be confusing to make sense of all the different weight-related words used by your WLS team. Here are some of the most common ones you're likely to hear, or have probably heard:

- Body mass index (BMI);
- Ideal/normal body weight;
- Percent excess weight loss (%EWL);
- Expected weight;
- Best weight.

Body mass index (BMI)
BMI is a simple, albeit outdated, calculation that measures the relationship between your height and weight.

$$BMI = kg \text{ of body weight}/(\text{height in m})^2$$

BMI classifies people as either underweight, normal weight, overweight, or obese. We typically discourage our patients from calculating their BMI because we don't feel that it's an appropriate marker of their true health or success.

Generally speaking, people who are classified as either overweight or obese are at a higher risk of developing weight-related health conditions such as diabetes, high blood pressure, and heart disease. Similarly, there's also health risks associated with being classified as underweight, such as poor bone health and malnutrition. For these reasons, BMI is often used to study large groups of people or populations for health research.

However BMI isn't perfectly accurate at predicting the health of everyone, which is why it's typically not recommended to use for individuals. We have many patients who classify as overweight or obese using BMI one year after WLS, despite achieving good success and who are healthy (i.e. no longer have diabetes nor high blood pressure, etc.).

The biggest flaw with this calculation is that it doesn't take into account how much of your weight is muscle versus how much is fat. For this reason, it often classifies healthy athletes as overweight or sometimes even obese! A bodybuilder might have a high BMI of 36 kg/m^2—classifying him as obese—but he has by no means the same health risks as a man who's the same age and height, doesn't exercise or eat properly, and who has a large abdomen.

Ideal, or 'normal', body weight
Many patients hope to achieve a 'normal' weight as per the BMI classification chart after surgery, but this often isn't a realistic expectation for most people. A better and more realistic goal would be to calculate the percent excess weight loss (%EWL) (see definition) you

are predicted to lose with WLS, and to discuss this expectation with your WLS team.

The bottom line: While BMI is still used by many health professionals, it's an outdated and inaccurate system for determining if you're a 'normal' weight, and whether your surgery has been a success.

Percent excess weight loss (% EWL)

This is the amount of excess (i.e. extra) weight that you've lost (or will lose) in relation to your ideal body weight. Remember that your ideal body weight is calculated as the higher end of what's considered a normal BMI. So for example, if you weigh 100 lbs more than your ideal body weight (IBW), and you lose 60 lbs with WLS, you've lost 60% of your *excess* weight (60 lbs / 100 lbs). Your WLS team can tell you what percent excess weight loss (%EWL) you've achieved at each visit.

The chart below compares the average percent excess weight loss for each WLS procedure:

WLS Procedure	Percent excess weight loss (% EWL)*
Gastric band	50%
Sleeve gastrectomy	60%
Gastric bypass (Roux-en-Y)	70%
Duodenal switch (DS)	80%

*Typically achieved at 12-18 months after surgery.

It's important to note that the percent excess weight you're predicted to lose is different for each surgery, and it's something to take into account when choosing your surgery.

It's also important to remember that you're not expected to lose 100% of your excess weight, and that few patients reach what's considered a normal BMI after surgery (i.e. lose 100% of their excess weight).

Remember, these percentages are an *estimation*. Some patients lose more than these predictions, some patients lose less. For a more tailored prediction of where you will stabilize after surgery, ask your WLS team what they predict your expected weight may be.

Percent weight loss (%WL) or percent total weight loss (%TWL)

This is a similar measurement to the percent excess weight loss (%EWL), however it counts the *total* weight loss instead of just the *excess* loss. Again, this is a calculation to help predict how much weight you'll lose based on what research shows is the average amount lost with each surgery.

For example, if you weighed 250 lbs before surgery and you lost 60 lbs with surgery, this means you've lost 24% (60 lbs / 250 lbs) of your total weight. It'll be a lower number than the percent excess weight loss (%EWL) even though the weight you've lost is the same. It is simply a different way of calculating the weight that you lose. Your WLS team can tell you what percent total weight you've lost at each visit.

'Expected' weight

Before your surgery, your WLS team should discuss with you your 'expected' weight, or the weight you're predicted to stabilize at around your first year after surgery. This number is based on several different factors, and it's *not* the amount of weight you hope to lose, but rather it's the amount you're predicted to lose with your surgery. This number is essentially an educated guess based on research and your WLS team's clinical experience. This number can also change over time as you lose weight, and it's different for everyone.

What factors help to predict your expected weight? Some of them include:

- Your starting weight;
- Which type of WLS you'll be having (i.e. %EWL);
- Your age and gender;
- Body frame size (e.g. small, medium, large);
- Your ability to be active after surgery (i.e. do you need a cane, walker, or wheelchair?);
- The medications you take;
- Any health issues you suffer from.

There are also lots of other factors that impact your weight loss journey that we cannot predict for prior to surgery. These factors include:

- Your genetics;
- Your metabolism;
- Your hormones;
- If you face complications after surgery;
- How closely you follow your team's eating plan and exercise recommendations.

Because of these factors, we can't guarantee what your expected weight will be, but your WLS team *can* give you a rough estimate of what you can expect after surgery.

After receiving their expected weight, many patients often say something along the lines of, "no way, I know I can lose more than that. I'll work extra hard, and lose more than the average patient. I'll be different."

More often than not, your WLS team will accurately predict your expected weight within 10 to 15 lbs, so it's important to accept the number your team gives you as your goal. This is something we cannot stress enough! Having realistic weight loss expectations is key to being satisfied with your weight loss journey. We often see patients who—in *our* eyes—have done excellent, but—in *their* eyes—are nowhere close to their personal, albeit unrealistic, weight loss goal. This disappointment can be easily avoided by having an open and honest conversation with your WLS team before undergoing surgery.

Best weight

Dr. Yoni Freedhoff and Dr. Arya Sharma, leaders in the field of obesity awareness, define the concept of *best weight*:

> *"A patient's best weight is … the healthiest lifestyle a patient can realistically enjoy, not the healthiest lifestyle a patient can tolerate….There comes a point when a person cannot eat less or exercise more and still like their life. The weight they attain while still liking their life is thus their "best" weight…".*
>
> - Freedhoff, Y. & Sharma, A. (2010). Best Weight: A Practical Guide to Office-Based Obesity Management. Canadian Obesity Network - Réseau canadien en obésité (CON-RCO).

Your best weight is:

- A weight you feel healthy at if you were to ignore the number on the scale;
- A weight where you're paying attention to what you're putting into your body, but you're not obsessing over calories and experiencing feelings of guilt;
- A weight where you are moving your body as often as you can;

- A weight where your health is the best it's been in previous years;
- A weight that you only realise you have reached once you get there.

Your best weight is *not*:

- Determined by your BMI;
- Necessarily a number you'd like to see;
- What an online forum thinks you should weigh;
- Can't be calculated or promised to you before you get there.

What is 'normal' weight loss after WLS?

After weight loss surgery, everyone loses weight at a different rate, which makes it *really* hard to define what 'normal' weight loss is. However it's important to have some average weight loss numbers in mind to reassure yourself that you are on track. For example, many patients who undergo bariatric surgery (also known as weight loss surgery, and commonly abbreviated to WLS) anticipate losing 30 to 50 lbs per month after the surgery—which rarely occurs—and can become discouraged when this isn't the case for them.

In our experience, the *average* patient (i.e. starting at a weight of 200-300 lbs) loses roughly three to five pounds per week, or 10-15 lbs per month during the first three months following their surgery, after which it's normal for the rate of weight loss to start slowing down. Most patients will lose weight up until 12 months after surgery, but it can actually range anywhere from nine to even 15 months.

The rate of weight loss varies for multiple reasons, and can even be a matter of perspective. For instance, if you have 100 lbs to lose then you're likely to lose more pounds per week than someone who has 50 lbs to lose. Meaning that, if you have less weight to lose, you may not be hitting the average of 10-15 lbs lost per month, but could very well be on track with your progress.

Here's a graph of a patient tracking their progress over the first 12 months after surgery:

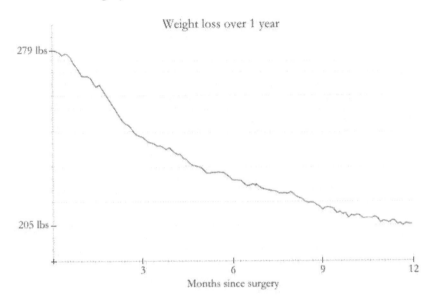

There are a couple key things to notice:

1. The rate of weight loss is quickest in the first few months after surgery (i.e. the line is steeper at the top).

2. The rate of weight loss begins to slow down around the ninth month, and stops at roughly 12 months (i.e. the line is flattening out at nine months and is flat by 12 months, meaning the patient's weight is now stable). This is likely the patient's best weight (we discussed the concept of best weight a few pages back).

3. Did you notice that the weight loss line over the course of the 12 months is never perfectly straight? Weight loss is *never*

constant. In tracking your own weight, you may notice that there are small day to day fluctuations and you may even *gain* one to two lbs every once in a while. So remember to take a step back and look at the graph as a whole, and remind yourself of the overall downward trend.

4. It's not easy to see on the graph, but this patient experienced a plateau (no weight loss) during week four. Plateaus, or stalls, can be super frustrating, we know! So it's important to know that plateaus are a normal part of the weight loss process, especially during the first couple months after surgery.

Why am I not losing weight? A conversation about plateaus/stalls.

It can be frustrating to undergo WLS and find yourself staying the same weight for a few weeks, or even months, after surgery. *What am I doing wrong? Is the surgery not working? Is my scale broken?* These are all normal thoughts to have, but relax. There's no need to panic.

A stable weight for more than a week is called a 'plateau' or a 'stall', and is simply your body's way of adjusting to your weight loss. Some plateaus resolve with rapid weight loss, as if to make up for the stall, while others simply resume the same rate of weight loss as before. Not all patients hit plateaus or stalls but, from our experience, the faster your weight loss is in the weeks after surgery the more likely you are to experience a plateau.

To understand if your plateau is simply a normal part of the weight loss process, or if it's related to your eating habits, ask yourself the following questions:

- Did I start drinking sugar-sweetened beverages (e.g. juice, sweetened coffees, sodas, etc.) that I wasn't drinking before my plateau, or stall, started?
- Am I drinking and eating at the same time?
- Have I started grazing (i.e. picking/nibbling) on food during the day?
- Am I having a hard time meeting my protein needs?

If you answer no to all of these questions, then you're experiencing a normal weight plateau which should end soon.

I gained one to two pounds since yesterday, what am I doing wrong?

Sunday	Monday	Tuesday	Wednesday	Thursday	Friday	Saturday
-	1 240.0 lbs	2 240.5 lbs	3 242.5 lbs	4 241.5 lbs	5 241.5 lbs	6 237.0 lbs
7 238.0 lbs	8 238.5 lbs	9 239.5 lbs	10 239.0 lbs	11 237.0 lbs	12 234.5 lbs	13 235.0 lbs
14 236.5 lbs	15 237.0 lbs	16 237.0 lbs	17 235.5 lbs	18 234.5 lbs	19 234.5 lbs	20 234.1 lbs

The calendar above is from an actual patient. Notice the daily fluctuations in weight?

If we look *across* the calendar or compare day to day (e.g. the 1st to 3rd) it looks like the patient has gained weight (e.g. +2.5 lbs)! However, if we look *down* the calendar or compare week to week (e.g. the 1st, 8th, and 15th) we can clearly see that the patient has lost weight (e.g. -3 lbs).

For this reason, we recommend that you weigh yourself only 1-2 times per week. Seeing day to day fluctuations can be very discouraging and confusing.

What is causing these fluctuations?

When your weight fluctuates from one day to the next, it's related to several factors, including:

- Drinking fluids before getting on the scale;
- Having had a meal or snack within the past few hours;
- Constipation;
- Hormonal changes related to menstruation;
- Fluid shifts possibly related to hypertension or fluid retention.

Overeating or eating too many calories can lead to weight gain, but did you know that it takes about 3500 calories more than what you're already consuming to gain one pound of fat? Before you worry, ask yourself if you ate an extra 3500 calories the day before? If the answer is no, then the weight increase isn't from gaining fat and likely due to one of the reasons listed above. Although this is an oversimplified example, we hope you can see what we are trying to get at.

The bottom line: We recommend that you weigh yourself only 1-2 times a week. This will prevent you from becoming frustrated by day to day fluctuations.

My weight has slowly been increasing. I've gained one to two pounds over the past week/month. What's happening?

Unlike the previous question, if you're consistently gaining weight from one week to the next and it continues for four to five weeks, then it's time to re-evaluate your habits.

Ask yourself the following questions:

1. Am I exercising to the point where I'm breaking a sweat and weight training several times a week? If yes, proceed to question two. If not, jump ahead to question three.

2. Although I've gained a small amount of weight, has my body clearly changed over the past 4-5 weeks (e.g. clothes fit looser, arms or legs have more definition, etc.)? If yes, this is still a sign of fat loss. If your body weight is increasing very slowly but your shape is slimming down, you're likely building muscle. Start keeping track of your pant size and what belt hole you're using since changes in body shape are more telling than the numbers on the scale.

3. Have you added something to your diet that wasn't there a few months ago (like juice, soda, sweetened drinks, alcohol, chips, or sweets)? If yes, then remember when we pointed out that it takes an extra 3500 calories to put on one pound of weight? If you added one chocolate bar (350 calories) and a bottle of juice to your day (150 calories), you wouldn't see a change in your weight immediately. But if you ate these foods every single day, you'd see a change by the end of the week. Similarly, if you

added these foods in every other day, you'd see an increase in your weight within two weeks.

Now, if you only had surgery less than six months ago, you wouldn't necessarily see an increase in your weight (e.g. after adding a daily chocolate bar and juice), but rather you'd see a significant slowdown in your weight loss. However, if you're approaching your one year anniversary, then you may start to see an increase in your weight if you haven't kept up the recommended habits. Now's the time to start correcting them, otherwise these habits will lead to more weight gain. Speak with your WLS dietitian to find a balance that works for you.

Why are my friends losing more weight than me?

Please, please, *please* do not compare your weight loss journey to that of others. It's not fair to yourself and all the hard work that you've put into this process. Success looks and feels different for everyone. Don't let your success be defined by someone else's number on a scale. There are five main reasons why some patients lose more than others.

1. Starting weight
The higher your starting weight, the greater number of pounds you'll lose. For example, someone who weighs 350 lbs will lose more weight with the same surgery and habits than someone who weighs 250 lbs. This is why you'll hear your WLS team talk about your weight loss in terms of your percent excess weight loss (%EWL). To use the same example, if both of these patients lost 60% of their excess weight and, for the sake of this example assume that both patients are the same height (5 feet 8 inches), the 350 lbs patient will lose 111 lbs while the

250 lbs patient will lose 51 lbs. Both are excellent and appropriate weight losses.

The bottom line: Percent excess weight loss (%EWL) is more appropriate as a measure of weight loss than the number of pounds shed.

2. Habits before surgery

Typically, the more you eat or the worse your eating habits were before surgery, the more weight you'll lose with WLS. For example, if two patients are the same height and starting weight, but one is eating 6,000 calories a day before surgery, while the other is eating 2,500 calories, the one consuming more will likely lose more weight, assuming they both have the same good eating habits after surgery.

The bottom line: The bigger the change in habits, the larger the change in weight.

3. Metabolism

Your metabolism is essentially how efficient your body is at processing what you feed it. The faster your metabolism, the more calories you burn per day. Alternatively, the slower your metabolism is the fewer calories you burn per day. So if we have two patients who have had WLS who are identical in every way except for their metabolisms, and we feed them both 1250 calories per day, they won't lose the same amount of weight. Theoretically, the person with the faster metabolism will lose more weight than the person with the slower metabolism.

Unfortunately, there's nothing you can do to significantly speed up your metabolism, despite what ads for teas, pills, drinks, and a million other products promise.

4. Current habits

It's also possible that your friends who are losing more weight are eating better and exercising more often than you. Remember that you only see how they behave in public, you don't see the other 80% of their hard work behind closed doors.

5. Type of surgery

Patients who've had gastric bypass will normally lose a higher percentage of their weight than patients who've had a sleeve gastrectomy. Similarly, those who undergo the duodenal switch will lose a higher percentage of weight than those who have undergone gastric bypass. The differences in weight loss between the surgeries are due to how much malabsorption there is with each WLS procedure.

6. Everything else

Medications, hormones, age, gender, genetics, and all of those other factors that you have little to no control over, can affect your weight loss. You need to accept that there are many things affecting your weight that, for better or worse, you can't change.

Remember, your weight loss is a personal journey *not* a public competition. Watch out for support groups and forums that foster competition instead of genuine support. Surround yourself with genuine people who truly care about you and your success.

I'm struggling to accept my best weight.

Many patients have unrealistic expectations for their weight loss journey, especially when it comes to their best weight. If you're still in the planning stages of your surgery, make sure you discuss your expectations with your WLS team. It's important to have realistic goals to prevent disappointment in the long run.

If you get frustrated or disappointed with your weight loss, here are some points to remember:

The journey

Many of our patients are so busy looking forward, and focusing on what they haven't achieved, that they forget to celebrate how far they've come. How has your relationship with food changed? How do you feel? How's your energy level? Are you out of breath less often? Do your clothes feel better on you? Be proud of yourself and all the healthy changes you've made.

What are you searching for?

Sometimes patients associate a specific weight with a time in their life in which they were happier, more confident, had more friends… the list goes on and on. Two important questions to consider are: What will you gain at your goal weight that you don't have now? What is it that you're longing for?

Sit with these feelings and be as honest as possible with yourself. Chances are you're looking for something that a number on the scale can't give you.

WLS is a medical surgery, not a cosmetic one

There are so many numbers *other* than those on the scale that change following WLS, and it's important to consider how your overall health has improved. How's your blood sugar? Your blood pressure? Your cholesterol? Your waist circumference? Do you take fewer pills per day? Fewer doctor's appointments per year? The ultimate goal of WLS is to improve your overall health and quality of life.

Celebrate your victories!

Would you be where you are today without your surgery? We challenge you to make a list of all the little things you couldn't do before your surgery that you now can. For example, can you cross your legs? Fit comfortably in a chair at the theatre? Enjoy roller coasters at theme parks?

Acceptance

For many of our patients, the process of acceptance takes time, often years. Remind yourself of the definition of best weight, and the importance it serves following WLS. You'll never be truly happy without reaching this stage of acceptance. If you need help, working with a psychologist might be a good place to start.

We highly recommend watching the documentary *Embrace* (2016), which offers a fabulous perspective on the topics of weight and size acceptance.

CHAPTER 2:

Tolerance Issues

Nausea and vomiting

Nausea and vomiting are common in the first few weeks after surgery. They improve with time.

The most common reasons for nausea are:

- Eating or drinking too quickly, or swallowing too much food or liquid at once;
- Not drinking enough liquids (dehydration);
- Side effects from the anesthesia and/or medication.

The most common reasons for vomiting are:

- Eating or drinking too quickly, or swallowing too much food or liquid at once,
- Not chewing enough (remember that bites of food should be no bigger than the size of your pinky fingernail);
- Drinking and eating at the same time;
- Eating when stressed or when multitasking;
- Progressing textures too quickly (i.e. trying regular texture foods when you should still be on purees).

Note: If you're on the puree menu and are experiencing a lot of nausea and/or vomiting, it could be because your homemade purees are too thick. Try thinning your purees by adding more liquid (like broth or milk). Your purees should not have any chunks in them and should be smooth.

Why doesn't food taste the same anymore?

After surgery, some patients claim food doesn't taste the same to them, specifically sweet tasting, oily, and greasy foods, as well as specific foods like milk, meat, eggs, and coffee. These taste changes seem to last anywhere from a few weeks to a few months and are likely due to the anesthesia and/or gut hormone changes that happen after surgery.

Taste changes usually improve with time, but for the time being, here are some tips to help you out:

- Instead of fruit yogurt, choose plain yogurt;
- If milk doesn't taste right, choose plain soymilk;
- Avoid added-sugars to tea and coffee;
- Instead of sweetened protein powder or protein shakes, choose plain/unflavoured protein powder and add it to a vegetable, chicken, or beef broth;
- Use a small amount of cooking oil when preparing food;
- If chicken, fish or meat doesn't taste right, flavour it with some lemon or vinegar and a little bit of salt;
- Choose other protein options such as tofu, legumes (lentils, chickpeas, red/black beans), and cheese.

If the smell of food turns you off eating or makes you queasy, here are some additional suggestions to follow:

- Have someone else cook for you if possible and stay out of the kitchen while food is cooking;

- Prepare cold meals (e.g. ham and cheese sandwich, legume salad, cottage cheese with fruit, hard boiled eggs, etc.) as cold foods have less of an odour;
- Have leftovers cold and avoid heating them up in the microwave.

Foods blocking or getting stuck

After WLS, it is common to experience problems 'tolerating' your food, especially in the first couple of months after surgery. What do we mean when we use the phrase 'poor tolerance'? Tolerance issues are most often described as when bites of food 'block' or feel like they're stuck in your esophagus after you swallow. It may feel like the food didn't make it to your stomach, like it's lodged mid-chest or higher. Although uncomfortable, sometimes to the point of intense pain, this issue isn't typically harmful to your new stomach.

What should you do when this happens? Some patients feel the need to bring the food back up (i.e. vomit), while others simply wait for the food to eventually pass. Tolerance issues can be very scary and uncomfortable, just remember to breathe through them.

Tolerance issues improve with time. It takes most patients three to six months to tolerate all foods, and even then, it is normal to have a couple of foods that just don't agree with you. When a food doesn't agree with you for the first time, either choose to avoid it for a couple of weeks, try cooking it a different way, take smaller bites next time, or simply eat slower. Getting used to the new sensations involved in eating after WLS takes practice.

What is abnormal food tolerance and when should I contact my WLS team?

Anything new takes some getting used to, so it's normal that eating may feel differently following WLS. It's normal to have a bit of nausea and some discomfort as you get to know the limits of your new stomach and as you test new food textures and new types of food. Eating after surgery is a new experience and requires some trial and error. However, it's important to know the difference between normal tolerance and abnormal tolerance.

If you are experiencing any of the following, you should contact your WLS team as soon as possible:

- Difficulty swallowing small sips of liquid (it's normal in the weeks following surgery to have *some* discomfort when swallowing plain water, but it's abnormal for the liquid to not go down or to vomit water regularly);
- Vomiting most of your meals and snacks.

When you contact your WLS team about your difficulty tolerating food and/or liquids, they will try to assess if this is related to:

- The type of food or drink you're having;
- If you're eating too quickly or taking gulps of liquids instead of sips;
- If your symptoms are due to irritation in your stomach or throat;
- If your symptoms are due to a stricture or stenosis.

Strictures and stenoses are complications that can occur after surgery and are most commonly associated with the gastric bypass and the gastric band, respectively. These complications are a result of either a narrowing of the new connection between your stomach and your small intestine (after a gastric bypass), or a narrowing created by the gastric band that is either too tight or is out of place. Stenoses and strictures can make it difficult to tolerate thick liquids, purees, and *especially* solid foods. Symptoms typically show up in the first three weeks after a gastric bypass or after an adjustment to your gastric band. These complications are manageable, but without having the problem fixed your symptoms likely won't improve. Once the stenosis or stricture is treated, you'll be able to drink and eat more comfortably almost immediately. Your WLS team will be able to discuss treatment options with you and answer all of your questions.

What foods are difficult to tolerate after surgery?

When you start eating solid foods again, usually six to seven weeks after surgery, depending on the recommendations of your WLS team, it's important to transition slowly. You shouldn't be jumping from purees one day to barbecued steak the next! Foods that are soft and moist are *always* tolerated better and with every passing month, your tolerance will improve. By about six months after surgery you should be able to eat most foods again, and if there are some that still give you trouble, remember not to worry; it's common to have a couple of foods that will always be tough to tolerate. Unfortunately, this is a reality after WLS.

The following is a list of the most common foods that can be difficult to tolerate after WLS. We've also included some tips on how to make them easier to tolerate.

Food	Explanation	Tips
Water	The cold temperature or drinking too much at once can cause issues after surgery. The experience of swallowing water after surgery is often described as swallowing a rock.	⇨ Add a small amount of juice, or a zero calorie water enhancer. ⇨ Experiment with warm and room temperature liquids. ⇨ Try herbal tea or decaf coffee instead. ⇨ Try bottled spring water. ⇨ Take smaller sips (e.g. 1/2 tsp at a time) and wait longer between sips.

Meat and fish (baked or barbecued)	Too tough and dried out.	⇨ Bake your meats and fish in sauce or broth in the oven. Cover with tinfoil to lock in the moisture. ⇨ Use dipping sauces for added moisture (e.g. ketchup, salsa, etc.). ⇨ Choose ground meats cooked in sauce (i.e. meat sauce, chili). Ground meats are easier to digest because they're already minced into small pieces. ⇨ Moisten canned tuna with a small amount of mayo. ⇨ Avoid barbecuing. Choose moist cooking methods. ⇨ Tenderize tough cuts of meat. ⇨ Add sauce or broth when reheating leftovers in the microwave.

Fresh breads	Too doughy. They often clump when swallowed due to the gluten.	⇨ Slice them and toast them. ⇨ Try pitas, tortillas, or crackers instead. ⇨ Consider gluten-free alternatives.
Pasta and rice	Too doughy. Like breads, they often clump when swallowed.	⇨ Try whole grain or gluten-free pasta. ⇨ Try smaller pastas like macaroni instead of long spaghetti noodles ⇨ Try tofu pasta. ⇨ Try overcooking pastas and add extra water when cooking rice.
Eggs	The texture can feel uncomfortable in the stomach, usually due to the yolk being too dry or thick. Fried eggs tend to be the trickiest type of prepared eggs.	⇨ Try soft boiled eggs or egg salad (add mayo). ⇨ Try an omelette with milk whisked in. ⇨ If omelettes and soft boiled eggs fail, try an egg white omelette.

Raw vegetables and fruit	Fibrous skins are difficult to chew well.	⇨ Remove any tough parts (i.e. the skin on cucumbers and apples). ⇨ Cook your fruits and vegetables to break down some of the fibre.
Stringy or tough fruits and vegetables (e.g. celery, artichokes, pineapple, oranges, corn, and asparagus)	Difficult to chew well.	⇨ Cook these foods to help breakdown some of the fibre. ⇨ Cut these foods against the fibre into small pieces. ⇨ Chew extra well!

One sure way to improve the tolerance of *all* of your foods is to take small bites and to slow down. This is something that we can't stress enough! Almost all foods will block if you take large bites and swallow quickly. If you described yourself as a fast eater before surgery, this is going to be a daily challenge for you. Try eating with your non-dominant hand or with chopsticks!

How do you know if you're chewing enough? A good goal is to chew all of your food until it's puree in your mouth, wait 15-30 seconds between bites, and make sure your meal takes 20-30 minutes to have one cup of food. Remember that digestion starts in the mouth!

Do I need to avoid nuts and seeds?

Many patients avoid nuts and seeds for months after surgery because they're afraid they won't be able to tolerate them. This isn't necessary. Although they might seem scary because of how crunchy and dry they are, the majority of patients digest nuts and seeds really well. Remember that a snack portion of nuts and seeds equals a quarter cup.

Our list of well tolerated soft solids

So you're finally ready to start solid or regular texture foods. This can be a scary transition and you've likely heard horror stories of patients having a really tough time, being constantly nauseous, and experiencing a lot of vomiting. But this isn't the majority of patients, and it doesn't have to be your story if you follow our tips.

The following is a list of easy to digest high protein foods that are usually well tolerated:

- Chili (vegetarian or with meat);
- Ground meat cooked in sauce;
- Moist meatloaf or meatballs;
- Shepherd's pie (without corn) served with ketchup;
- Thick chickpea, bean, or lentil stew;
- Fish cooked in broth;
- Tuna with a small amount of mayo;
- Egg salad made with a small amount of mayo eaten with crackers;
- Tofu cooked in sauce.

Some other tips include:

- Start with cooked vegetables as raw vegetables are harder to digest in the beginning;
- Start with easy to digest fruits (e.g. peeled pear, half a banana, peeled apple, berries, and melons) and remove the skin and other tough parts.

If you can't tolerate a food, wait another week before trying it again.

And remember: If you're not tolerating the puree menu that your WLS team has instructed you to follow (i.e. you are experiencing nausea and/or vomiting regularly), then you're not ready to transition to soft solids. Stay on purees for another week and call your WLS dietitian for more advice.

What foods can I never eat again after surgery?

'Never' is a strong word. 'Never' is a word commonly used by chronic dieters who follow the all or nothing approach, meaning you're either strictly on a diet or off a diet. There's no middle ground. But in our opinion there isn't any food that you're *never* allowed after surgery. However, there *are* foods that can be problematic after WLS for a few reasons.

Sweets
Aside from the obvious fact that sweets (e.g. candy, cookies, chocolate, pastries, ice cream, etc.) are high in both calories and sugar, with little to no nutritional benefits, they also can cause dumping syndrome after

a gastric bypass. For these reasons, sweets should be consumed in smaller portions and eaten less often.

High fat, oily, greasy foods

Given the high calorie content of deep fried and greasy foods, every bite eaten is higher in calories. If you eat fried foods regularly, you may lose weight in the first few months after surgery because you're eating less of it, but in a year's time you may not reach your expected weight because you're consuming more calories than if you were not eating fried food.

If you have a duodenal switch, high fat greasy foods may lead to what's called steatorrhea, or oily and frequent stools. This is because your body can't absorb fat like it used to, which causes you to run to the washroom after you have eaten a high fat meal. High fat, oily, and greasy foods should be consumed in smaller portions and eaten less often.

Tough foods

This includes tough meats like beef and pork. Most patients have difficulty eating these foods to start with, but their tolerance can improve over the first year following WLS. These foods do not need to be avoided, instead you should simply re-try them every few weeks to see if your tolerance for them has improved. It's normal to tolerate some cuts of these meats and not others (for instance, it's possible that ground beef in tomato sauce passes well but a BBQ steak doesn't). This has to do with how tough/tender and how dry/moist the meat is. As previously mentioned, the cooking method has a lot to do with this.

Fibrous foods

These foods can include fresh celery stalks, artichokes, asparagus, pineapple, and popcorn. While some WLS centres suggest that you no longer eat these foods, there's no real evidence to justify this. From our experience, as long as you tolerated these foods (i.e. you have no discomfort after eating them), they're fine to consume.

Doughy sticky foods
This includes bread, rice, and pasta. These foods don't need to be avoided, however, they're commonly poorly tolerated, meaning that most patients feel discomfort or a blocking sensation after eating them, or they may vomit.

Caffeine
Foods and drinks that are high in caffeine, like coffee and energy drinks, should be limited. General recommendations advise that caffeine be limited between 300 mg to 400 mg, or two to three eight-ounce cups of coffee every day. More than this can begin causing health concerns like sleeping problems, irritability, stomach irritation, and nervousness. A high intake of caffeine, more than 300 mg of caffeine per day, can begin to dehydrate the body. Since it's already difficult for most to drink enough water on a daily basis (1.5 to 2 L/day), a high intake of caffeine may increase the risk of dehydration.

Alcohol
Alcoholic drinks—including beer, wine, spirits, and mixed beverages—can irritate your stomach and intestines. It's recommended to wait until the rapid weight loss has slowed down, or at least six months after surgery to reintroduce alcohol. Remember that you shouldn't drink and eat at the same time.

Carbonated beverages
Fizzy drinks are discouraged after surgery because it's believed that the carbonation can stretch the stomach over time. They are also not recommended because non-diet drinks contain extra calories which can lead you to regain weight. Early on after surgery, the carbonation in these beverages can lead you to feel pain and discomfort due to the gas

building up in your small stomach. While it's unlikely that only a few sips of a carbonated drink will do you any harm, the true question is will a few sips of a carbonated beverage result in cravings leading you to drink more of it? Will the taste of your favourite soda increase your desire for junk food or takeout?

Only you know if this was a problem for you before surgery and, if it was, the cravings aren't simply going to disappear after surgery. Relapsing is always possible, so we suggest treating any problem foods (foods you have a serious weakness for) like you would alcohol addiction: avoid it at all cost, no matter how difficult it can be, and seek support.

How can I tenderize my meats and what cuts are better tolerated?

A common problem faced after surgery is difficulty tolerating meats. While this is often caused by taking bites that are too big (i.e. bigger than your pinky fingernail) and not chewing well enough, difficulty tolerating meats can also be caused because the cut of meat is too tough or wasn't cooked properly.

Here are our top tips for improving the tolerance and digestibility of your meats:

- Choose tender cuts of meat (these include ground meats, tenderloin [filet mignon], top blade [flat iron], top loin steak, sirloin, porterhouse steak, and all poultry [especially chicken thighs and drumsticks]), and avoid tough cuts (like stewing beef, brisket, top and bottom round, and chuck roast);

- Cook meats until *just* done (the trick to not overcooking meats is to use a meat thermometer when cooking to measure their internal temperature. Overcooking certain cuts of meat will make naturally tender cuts tough and dry);

- Slow cook meats at low temperatures for a longer period of time (a slow-cooker makes a great investment after surgery);

- If your budget allows, pick meats with more marbling (thin white lines of fat within meat);

- Manually tenderize your meats with a kitchen mallet before cooking them as it helps to break down the tough muscle fibres which your new stomach has a hard time digesting;

- Naturally tenderize your meats by using enzymes found in fruit. Add one to two tablespoons of pureed lemon, kiwi, pineapple, or papaya in your marinade and let sit overnight for best results;

- Naturally tenderize meats using a marinade that contains vinegar as they're naturally acidic and help denature (or breakdown) the protein found in meat (let them marinate overnight for best results);

- Chemically tenderize your meats using baking soda (yes, that little box that you use to remove odours from your fridge!) by slicing up your meat into thin slices (about ¼" thick), mixing in one to two teaspoons of baking soda to coat the meat, and letting it sit for 15 minutes. Rinse with water and then stir-fry with a sauce.

I overcooked my meat and now it's too tough. How can I salvage it?

You can try to salvage already cooked meat by cutting it into thin pieces and cooking it in a pan or in the oven with enough broth to cover it. Cover the pan or pot with aluminum foil, or with a pan cover, and cook it for 30 to 60 minutes (or longer), while checking every 30 minutes to test the meat for tenderness.

Why do certain foods go down one day, but not the next?

Generally, there are a few reasons this occurs, including:

Cooking methods
If you tolerated a saucy chicken pot-pie, it doesn't mean roast chicken will go down just as comfortably. Dry methods of cooking (like broiling, roasting, grilling, and pan-frying) tend to be more difficult to tolerate. Moist cooking methods on the other hand (like steaming, braising, stewing, simmering, poaching) that involve liquids or a sauce are typically better tolerated. Also, be careful when microwaving, as the process of reheating foods can dry them out. A good way to keep the moisture in is by resting the lid on the container (not sealed) and stir after each minute until ready. If you're reheating dry foods, remember to sprinkle in some water, broth, tomato juice, milk, or low fat gravy to add additional moisture.

Mechanical reasons
Mechanical reasons like not chewing well enough and taking large bites. You should always be sure to cut your food into small pieces—as small

as your pinky fingernail to start—and chew your food until it's puree in your mouth before swallowing. Remember that digestion starts in the mouth!

Emotional stress and anxiety

Emotional stress and anxiety can tighten the upper digestive system which makes food more difficult to tolerate. Do you find you eat more comfortably at home or on the weekends compared to at work? If so, your tolerance issues could be related to stress or anxiety. Always be sure to eat in a calm environment and start your meals by taking a few deep breaths to relax yourself and decompress. Some patients feel more comfortable eating alone at first (i.e. in their office instead of in the cafeteria).

Eating while multitasking!

When you are eating, you should *only* be eating. We know that this is a tough one to practice, but eating while driving, watching TV, cleaning, working through lunch, etc. can distract you from taking small bites and chewing well. Do your best to eliminate distractions during meal times. If you choose to eat lunch in your office, mute the volume on your computer and turn off the monitor so you're not tempted to check your email between bites.

Posture

It sounds silly to discuss, but it's true; poor posture can negatively affect digestion. If you are eating while slouched, reclined on the couch, or awkwardly propped up on pillows in bed, chances are that you will experience some tolerance issues. When you are eating, you should ideally be sitting in a chair pulled close to the table with your bottom as far back as possible and with your back nice and straight. Eating at the table in your kitchen or dining room will also give your meals and snacks more structure. Generally speaking, it's a good habit to limit eating to only the kitchen and dining room.

Heartburn

Heartburn, also known as acid reflux, is often described as a burning feeling in your chest. Heartburn occurs when the acid from your stomach comes up into your esophagus, which is the tube connecting your mouth to your stomach. Not only is this uncomfortable and can lead to feeling nauseated or unwell, but it's also damaging to the sensitive tissue of your esophagus. Over time, and if left untreated, it can cause serious damage and increases your risk of developing stomach ulcers and cancer of the esophagus. Chronic heartburn is called gastroesophageal reflux disease or GERD.

Heartburn isn't a symptom to take lightly or ignore. It's normal to have a bit of heartburn in the weeks after surgery, however, it's important to resolve longer term heartburn by following the tips listed below or with medication as recommended by your WLS team.

Some tips for improving heartburn include:

- Avoid lying down immediately after eating, wait at least 45 minutes before reclining;
- Avoid eating 2-3 hours before you go to sleep;
- Avoid overeating;
- Eat slowly and chew your food well;
- Avoid foods high in fat and sugar;
- Avoid spicy foods;
- Quit smoking;
- Avoid tight clothing;
- Try over the counter antacids for the occasional heartburn, and be sure to ask your pharmacist for help choosing the right one.

Food triggers are different for everyone. Try tracking the severity of your heartburn symptoms by adding another column into your food journal to see if you can find links between specific foods and your symptoms.

Pay special attention to the following foods, as these foods are common triggers: high fat meals, high sugar meals, high fat dairy products, acidic foods (e.g. tomato products and citrus fruits), spices, garlic, onions, caffeinated products (especially before breakfast), and alcohol.

If your heartburn is severe or is occurring daily, we recommend you contact your WLS team for further advice. They'll likely prescribe a medication that will provide more complete, and faster relief.

What can I do to prevent or treat constipation while I'm still on the liquid/puree phase after surgery?

First off, are you truly constipated? It's normal to have less stool and fewer bowel movements in the first few weeks after surgery. If you're passing stool daily or easily, then perhaps you're not constipated, this is just your new or temporary cycle. However, if your bowel movements are only a few times a week, they're hard, and you need to force more than before WLS to pass them, you're constipated.

It's normal to experience constipation, especially in the first six to seven weeks after surgery, because you're not drinking much, you are eating significantly less and your diet is very low in fibre. Some medications and vitamins prescribed after surgery can also worsen constipation, but it's important to take your medication and vitamins as prescribed by your WLS team.

Here are some suggestions to help prevent and treat constipation:

- Drink approximately two litres (eight cups) of water daily. Try your best to sip on liquids all day, even if you're not thirsty. Warm fluids are also encouraged. If you're drinking enough, your urine will run clear by the end of the day and you should be urinating often;

- Include ¼ cup of pureed plums or ½ cup of prune juice daily;

- Increase the fibre in your diet (e.g. have pureed legume soups [chickpeas/beans/lentils] more often and add wheat germ/wheat bran/chia seeds/flax seeds, berries, spinach, high fibre cereals, and seeds [chia, flax, etc.] to your smoothies);

- Try taking a daily probiotic product (e.g. probiotic yogurt, kefir or a probiotic supplement in pill or liquid form). Probiotics are live bacteria that help keep your gut, or intestines, healthy (ask your WLS team or pharmacist for some examples);

- If you're already drinking at least two litres of fluids every day (or eight cups), try a powdered fibre supplement in small doses. Ask your WLS team or pharmacist for some examples, and always start with the lowest suggested dose—no matter how constipated you are—and increase as needed. Powdered fibre supplements are not recommended if you can't drink enough water because they can have the opposite effect and further constipate you;

- Walk 15 minutes daily after your meals to help get things moving;

- Place a footstool under your feet when sitting on the toilet to raise your knees above your hips as this position can help you to better empty your bowels;

- Ask your WLS team if they recommend you start a gentle over the counter laxative temporarily.

What can I do about constipation now that I've started solid foods after surgery?

Here are some additional tips for preventing and treating constipation if you're now on solid foods. Make sure to also incorporate the tips above as well.

- Add three tablespoons of psyllium fibre to your day by mixing it with your yogurt, oatmeal, to your smoothies, or add it to your favourite cereal. You can incorporate them at breakfast or as a snack. Psyllium fibre can also be found in certain cereals, so be sure to read the nutrition claims on the front of the packaging or in the ingredient list. It's most commonly found in bran or fibre-rich cereals, but be sure that it reads "contains psyllium" on the packaging;

- Legumes (which include chickpeas, lentils, beans, and edamame) tend to be very effective for relieving constipation due to their high fibre content so opt for a vegetarian chili, a thick lentil soup, a chickpea salad, or even a simple can of beans in tomato sauce;

- Choose whole grain products (e.g. bread, crackers, tortillas, whole wheat pasta, quinoa, etc.) with at least 3 grams of fibre per suggested serving;

- Have a snack of ¼ cup seeds (e.g. pumpkin, sunflower, etc.) or nuts (e.g. almonds, peanuts, soy nuts, etc.), and a fruit. On average, seeds and nuts pack 3 g of fibre per ¼ cup portion;

- Make sure you're having fruits and vegetables at every meal and snack. We're well aware that you can't fit a ton of these in with your limited portions, but every mouthful counts. Try a small handful of blueberries with breakfast, ½ a pear in your yogurt as a snack, or add five carrots to your lunch. The fibres found in fruits and vegetables will help get your system moving

The highest fibre fruits include: pears (with skin), apples (with skin), raspberries, bananas, and oranges/clementines/tangerines, and apricots. The highest fibre vegetables include: green peas, broccoli, spinach, Brussels sprouts, and carrots.

Note that high fibre foods can be difficult to digest. To improve the tolerance of the foods listed above, make sure to chew these foods really well and take 20-30 minutes for your meals, and 15 minutes for your snacks. If you've just recently transitioned to solid foods, you may not be ready to incorporate these tougher/high fibre options.

If your constipation isn't improving despite incorporating most of the above tips, if you've developed hemorrhoids, or if you are experiencing severe pain in passing stools, be sure to speak with your WLS team.

Is it possible to develop an intolerance to lactose after surgery?

Yes. It's possible, and pretty common, to develop an intolerance to lactose (a sugar found in milk and other dairy products) after surgery. Your body needs an enzyme called lactase to break down lactose in order to properly digest it. The lactase enzyme is produced at the start of the small intestine and in surgeries such as the gastric bypass and the duodenal switch, this part of the intestine is "bypassed". This means the lactose isn't able to join with the lactase enzyme, and as a result your body can no longer digest and absorb the lactose properly. While not everyone who has a gastric bypass or duodenal switch will experience lactose intolerance, it's definitely possible, particularly in patients who had a slight lactose intolerance before surgery. While lactose intolerance doesn't typically go away, most patients will be able to tolerate yogurt and cheese, as well as milk (in small amounts).

What are the symptoms of being lactose intolerant?

If you notice that you feel bloated, gassy, and/or experience diarrhea within a few minutes to an hour after consuming a dairy product (especially milk), you've likely developed an intolerance to lactose. Yogurt and cheese are often tolerated fairly well because these products contain lower amounts of lactose. You'll learn how much you can tolerate, through trial and error.

What should I do if I think I'm lactose intolerant?

If you think that you've developed lactose intolerance, you should avoid all lactose-containing foods for one week to see if your symptoms improve. To do this, choose lactose-free milk or soy milk, and choose only lactose-free products for your other dairy products (e.g. lactose-free yogurt and cheese). We don't recommend other alternative milk beverages like almond, cashew, rice, or coconut milk, etc. because these milks are very low in protein (as you'll see in the table on the next page).

Another option is to continue buying regular dairy products and take over-the-counter lactase pills or drops each time you have dairy. Lactaid pills contain enzymes that digest the lactose for you. Lactaid pills can be found at all pharmacies and purchased without a prescription.

The chart below compares the protein content of different milks:

Type of milk	Protein (in 1 cup)	Tips
Cow's milk or lactose-free milk	8 grams	Choose: 0% (skim), 1% or 2% M. F. (milk fat)
Soy milk	6 grams	Choose 'enriched' soy milk. This means it has added calcium, B vitamins and vitamin D.
Almond milk	1 gram	Choose cow's milk or soy milk for protein.
Cashew milk	< 1 gram	Choose cow's milk or soy milk for protein.
Rice milk	1 gram	Choose cow's milk or soy milk for protein.

Diarrhea

Diarrhea is less common after surgery than constipation, however it *can* happen. Diarrhea is defined as 3-5 liquid bowel movements per day.

Here is a list of the most common causes of diarrhea after WLS:

Lactose intolerance
Lactose intolerance, or not being able to digest the sugar (lactose) found in dairy products, can cause diarrhea. Does your diarrhea tend to be triggered by milk? If yes, you've likely developed an intolerance to lactose.

Antibiotics and medication
Are you taking antibiotics? If yes, this is most likely the cause of your diarrhea. Once you finish your dose of antibiotics your diarrhea should improve within 3-5 days. Ask your WLS team about taking a probiotic during and after your antibiotic treatment as this can help minimize the diarrhea and helps to replenish the good bacteria in your gut that the antibiotics 'killed'.

Another common reason for diarrhea is as a side effect from other medications that are commonly prescribed after surgery. Ask your WLS team or pharmacist if any of your new medications can cause this. And remember: never stop or change a medication without consulting a health professional first.

Dumping syndrome
Is your diarrhea triggered by sweet foods (e.g. juice, ice cream, candy, and chocolate)? If yes—and you've had a gastric bypass surgery—the cause of your diarrhea is likely dumping syndrome. More on this subject later.

Steatorrhea
This is oily or greasy stool. Is your diarrhea triggered by high fat foods (e.g. deep fried foods, sausages, bacon, etc.)? If yes—and you've had a duodenal switch —a high fat diet is likely the cause of your diarrhea.

Sugar alcohols
Sugar alcohols are natural sweeteners. They're found in low-sugar products, such as low/no sugar candies and chocolates. When you have too much of these types of products, the sugar alcohols can cause abdominal cramps, bloating, gas, and diarrhea. Sugar alcohols appear in the ingredient list of products under the following names: sorbitol, xylitol, maltitol, isomalt, lactitol and mannitol, just to name a few. Simply reducing your consumption of sugar alcohols will resolve your diarrhea in a couple of days.

Still experiencing diarrhea?

If you're experiencing diarrhea (i.e. more than 3-5 liquid bowel movements per day) during the first month after surgery and it doesn't appear to be related to any of the previous reasons, you should contact your WLS team as soon as possible. They'll likely ask you to provide a stool sample as it's possible you may have picked up a bacteria while you were in the hospital.

While you're experiencing diarrhea it's important to stay well hydrated. You need to increase the amount of water that you're drinking to replace the fluids you're losing. It's also suggested to rehydrate with electrolyte drinks (e.g. sports drinks).

Electrolyte drinks - Rehydrating after diarrhea or vomiting
Electrolyte drinks (or low sugar sports drinks) are strongly recommended if you're experiencing persistent diarrhea and/or vomiting. These drinks help to rehydrate you and quickly replace the electrolytes that you're flushing down the toilet! Carry an electrolyte

drink around with you all day in a water bottle and sip on it between meals and snacks.

Signs and symptoms of dehydration include:

- Headache;
- Dizziness or light-headedness;
- Fatigue.

Electrolyte and low sugar sports drinks can be found in grocery stores, corner stores, and pharmacies.

Lisa Kaouk & Monica Bashaw

CHAPTER 3:
Hunger & Appetite

What is the difference between hunger and appetite?

Both hunger and appetite encourage us to eat, but their triggers are very different.

Hunger is the physical *need* to eat.
It's usually felt as an emptiness in the stomach after having gone hours without eating. The easiest way to understand hunger is remembering the feeling you get when you've had to fast for a blood test or medical test. After 12 hours of fasting, your body is hungry and is counting down the time until you are allowed food again. This is often referred to as "true" hunger, because it's the real need to eat.

Appetite is the *desire* or the pure *want* to eat.
Think of a time that you weren't hungry, but someone walked into the room with something tasty and all of a sudden you wanted food. There was no emptiness in your stomach nor plan to eat before you saw the food. This is appetite. Appetite can be related to any number of things (e.g. nostalgia, boredom, feeling happy, stressed, or sad, etc.). Appetite is often referred to as 'head hunger' because it comes from the mind and not the stomach.

Learning when you're hungry vs when you have an appetite for something takes practice and may require help from a professional (e.g. a psychologist or a WLS dietitian).

Ask yourself the following questions the next time you're unsure if you're really truly hungry:

Tip 1
Keep a string, elastic, sticker, magnet, or anything that stands out to you on the handle of your fridge and pantry doors. Anytime you enter the kitchen to get some food, no matter if it's chips, cookies, a fruit, or some cheese, take the time to pause and ask yourself if you feel true hunger (the pit in your stomach) or head hunger (a desire to eat from boredom or emotions).

Tip 2
If you're still unsure if you're experiencing true hunger or not, offer yourself a food that you don't particularly like or one you feel neutral about, as if it were the only food left in your kitchen (e.g. mushrooms or green peppers). If—without—hesitation, you'd take the food, you're likely hungry. But if you pause and debate if you want it, you're likely not truly hungry.

Tip 3
Ask yourself if you're thirsty. We often confuse thirst for hunger. When was the last time you had a sip of water?

Tip 4
If you still can't figure it out, look at the clock and ask yourself when you last ate. If it's been 2.5-3 hours or more, then you're likely starting to feel true hunger. If it's been less than 2 hours, it's more likely appetite.

Tip 5

Ask yourself how you're hoping the food will make you *feel*. If the answer is simply: full, satisfied, or fuelled for the next couple of hours, then you're likely hungry. However, if you're hoping that eating or having a specific food will help you feel less anxious, less stressed, comforted, less lonely, less fidgety, less bored, etc., then you're eating for appetite. Working through these complex feelings can be tough. We recommend that you enlist the services of a local psychologist if you feel ready to heal your relationship with food.

Here is a simple and quick reference to look over the next time you're trying to determine if you're hungry or have an appetite:

Hunger:

- Symptoms include a growling stomach, feeling light-headed, having a headache and generally feeling weak;
- Gradually increases;
- Appears several hours after the last meal;
- Goes away with eating;
- Is satisfied by *any* type of food.
    - E.g. Jackie hates melon, but one day after work she was so hungry she ate a whole cup of melon because it was the only food left in the fridge.

Appetite:

- Triggers include emotions and boredom;
- Stimulated by seeing or smelling food;
- Begins suddenly;
- Starts at any time and can last for several minutes to several hours;
- Continues even after having eaten;

- Only satisfied with *specific* foods
  - I.e. Judy just ate her lunch and expressed to her colleagues that she felt full. Despite having a fruit in her bag, she still bought a chocolate bar from the vending machine at work. She knew she had food to eat but the fruit wasn't what she wanted: she craved chocolate.

Is it normal that I never feel hungry?

Before surgery, some patients say that they never felt hungry. This may be because the more body fat a person has, the more of the gut hormone 'leptin' is released in the body. This hormone stops you from feeling hungry.

After surgery, it's normal for some patients not to feel hungry because the stomach is very small and WLS patients have less of an ability to release the gut hormone 'ghrelin.' This hormone is what usually makes you feel hungry. Since you have less of it being released in your body after surgery, you won't feel hungry for some time (i.e. often up to 1-3 months after surgery). This will improve with time, but it's often a struggle in the first few months.

Do I need to eat even if I'm not hungry?

Yes! It's normal not to feel like eating after surgery, just like you may not feel like eating when you're sick. But it's important to eat well after WLS because your body needs to heal on the inside.

Skipping meals and snacks increases your risk of:

- Weight plateaus, since your weight loss may stall if you aren't properly fuelling your body;

- Hair loss, as a diet low in protein and low in calories increases your risk of hair shedding;

- Muscle loss, as a diet low in protein will increase your rate of muscle loss while you're losing weight (this has many negative health consequences, including slowing your metabolism, not to mention muscle mass is hard to gain back);

- Fatigue and general feeling of weakness, as fuelling your body is key to feeling energized;

- Constipation, since less food going in, means less to come out. Not to mention that low calorie diets are lower in fibre which helps keep you regular.

Some tips for eating regularly include:

- Setting a timer to remind yourself to eat every 2-3 hours throughout the day since you can't rely on your hunger to cue you at this time;

- Choosing liquid meal and snack options if you don't feel like eating since these types of options are often simple to prepare, lighter, and easier to digest (examples include: homemade smoothies, yogurt, protein shakes, soy milk, etc.).

How do I know when I'm full?

After surgery, some patients have difficulty recognizing when they're full after eating. Learning to listen and respond to your new stomach is a really important skill, one that takes time. The goal is to feel satisfied after a meal or snack, but not overly full like you would after a holiday meal. If you reach the point of being nauseated and/or vomiting, you have eaten too much. Next time eat less. Following the portions on the menus your WLS team has given or will give you is a good starting guide.

The best way to know if you're eating enough is to wait and see when you start feeling hungry again. If you feel hungry in 2 to 3 hours following your last meal, then you're probably eating enough. If however you feel true hunger within 1 to 2 hours, you probably need to eat a little bit more next time.

If you're comfortably able to eat more than one cup of food and don't feel satisfied, and it's been less than six months since you had WLS, you should discuss this with your WLS dietitian.

How do I know when to start and stop eating?

On the next page is a hunger and fullness scale. Your daily goal is to stay in the lighter zones (i.e. zones 4-7) and avoid the darkest zones. This is a challenging step towards a healthier relationship with food for many patients, but it's crucial to long term success.

Hunger & Fullness Scale

1 – STARVING: You are ravenous. You feel dizzy, weak and sick from hunger. You have a headache.

2 – FAMISHED: A lot of stomach growling. You are irritable and unable to concentrate. Low energy.

3 – VERY HUNGRY: Stomach is starting to growl. You are ready to eat an entire meal.

4 – HUNGRY: You are beginning to feel hungry. It is time to think about what to eat. You are not uncomfortable.

5 – NEUTRAL: You are neither hungry nor full.

6 – COMFORTABLE: You are beginning to feel satisfied. You are slightly full, but there is still room in your stomach.

7 – FULL: Your hunger is 100% satisfied. You do not need to eat more. You won't be hungry for several hours.

8 – VERY FULL: You have overdone it by several bites. You are slightly uncomfortable.

9 – OVER FULL: You are physically stuffed. You are very uncomfortable and nauseous. You need to loosen your belt.

10 – STUFFED: You ate way too much. The discomfort is painful. You feel sick, nauseous, and may vomit.

Avoiding the dark zones is all about listening to your internal cues and practising the daily eating guidelines that your WLS team has given you (i.e. eating regularly, eating slowly, eating mindfully, eating one cup maximum, including a protein source every time you eat, etc.).

You should stop eating *well* before you reach zones 8-10 and feel physically uncomfortable (i.e. nausea, heartburn, indigestion, belching, etc.). Your goal after surgery is to develop a new healthier relationship with your stomach. This means listening and reacting when your stomach is telling you to stop. For example, if ¾ cup of food makes you feel nauseous and uncomfortable, or even causes you to vomit, next time listen harder to your stomach and eat even slower as you reach the ½ cup mark to avoid entering the dark zones. Patients who are constantly pushing their stomachs past its comfortable limits are at a high risk for weight regain. If you're eating more than 1-1.5 cups of food per meal, you're defeating the purpose of the surgery.

Similarly, you want to avoid the darkest zones at the top of the scale (i.e. zones 1-3). This is often the end of the scale that we spend less time talking about, but it's equally important. If you're waiting until the point of starving to finally eat something, you've missed the mark and have waited too long to respond to your stomach's hunger signals. This is often when patients can't help but eat too fast because they're unbearably hungry, and as a result the food blocks.

For those of you who keep food journals (which we highly encourage!), a great exercise to incorporate into your journaling is to rank your hunger and fullness scores on a scale of one to ten before and after every meal and snack. Once you start to identify patterns, you can then adjust your meal and snack times and the protein content of your meals and snacks to keep your hunger more in control throughout the day. Your WLS dietitian can also help you with this.

A common pattern we see in our practice, is patients bouncing back and forth between the two ends of the scale and completely skipping over the middle section (i.e. zones 4-7). If you don't understand what we mean by this, read the scenario below. It may sound all too familiar to some of you!

You had a crazy day at work and there wasn't time for lunch. In the afternoon, around 3:00 p.m., when you thought you'd have time for a quick bite to eat, something came up and your boss needed you. By the time you left work, exhausted and famished (i.e. zone 2), all you could think about was getting home and eating. The drive home was a blur, your head was foggy from your blood sugar being so low. You opened the front door, dropped all of your work bags and immediately headed straight for the kitchen. You ate standing up in front of the fridge. You were eating fast, trying to fill the hole in your stomach. The next thing you know, maybe five minutes later, you were stuffed (i.e. zone 10). Physically uncomfortable and nauseous, you wandered into the living room and stretched out on the couch to try to relieve some of the discomfort.

If this is you, we highly recommend working with a WLS dietitian. This type of pattern will set you up to fail after surgery. These types of habits unfortunately don't change simply because you've had surgery.

Lisa Kaouk & Monica Bashaw

CHAPTER 4:

Water

Why is water difficult to swallow?

In the weeks after surgery, a lot of patients complain that it's difficult to drink plain water. They describe the experience as sips feelings heavy and each swallow hitting their stomach feeling like a rock. Other patients complain that they feel uneasy, nauseous, or like they have to burp to release a gassy feeling, but yet they can't.

We want to reassure you that this is very normal in the beginning. With time, your discomfort with water will improve.

In the meantime, try these tips to improve your tolerance to water:

- Add a flavour to your water with a dash of diluted juice or low calorie water enhancers;

- Experiment with the temperature of your water, since some patients swear they can only drink cold water, while others swear by warm water or room temperature water;

- Choose to hydrate instead with tea or decaf coffee;

- Chew on ice chips;

- Try using a straw, as some patients find that they can drink more water when they use one. Although using a straw is *super* controversial after surgery (try googling it!), we believe that if it doesn't cause you any discomfort then they're okay to use. The potential risk of using a straw to drink is that you often end up swallowing a lot of air, which can cause uncomfortable side effects such as burping, gas, and indigestion.

- Try bottled spring water. Due to the difference in mineral content, spring water is often tolerated better than mineral water and tap water.

How much water should I drink each day?

A good goal is to be drinking minimum 1.5-2.0 L/day, or 6-8 cups/day, of liquid per day to stay hydrated and healthy. Ideally, most of these liquids should be water and other low calorie beverages. Not drinking and eating at the same time is an extra challenge, but doesn't make it impossible. The key is to be sipping between your meals and snacks all day long. If you don't hydrate until the end of the day, reaching this goal is almost impossible.

In the days and first couple weeks after surgery, we are well aware that 1.5-2.0 L/day just isn't realistic, but it's still important to try your best. Remember that your ability to drink more water and other liquids will improve with each passing week. Also, don't forget that in the weeks following your surgery your meals and snacks are liquid or semi-liquid in texture, which is also helping to keep you hydrated.

Remember that all liquids (except alcohol) count towards this 1.5-2.0 L/day goal, including:

- Water;
- Tea;
- Homemade low-sugar/diluted iced tea;
- Milk;

- Soy milk;
- Smoothies;
- Protein drinks;
- Coffee*, regular and decaf;
- Diluted juice and diluted low sugar sports drinks.

*New research suggests that regular coffee is not as dehydrating (up to 400 mg of caffeine/day) as we once thought. We therefore count up to three cups of coffee towards your 1.5-2.0 L/day goal. However, it's important to limit your caffeine intake for other reasons.

Tips for drinking more water

For many of our patients, drinking enough water is a daily struggle.

Do any of the following comments sound familiar? *I just forget. I don't feel thirsty. I'm too busy. I feel limited by not drinking and eating at the same time. Water is boring!*

Here are our tips for getting in more water:

Make water more convenient by…

- Buying a fun new water bottle for work and home that gets you excited. Ideally, something colourful that catches your eye;

- Keeping a water bottle or water glass within arm's reach at all times, regardless of where you are (e.g. at work, in the car, on the couch, in bed, etc.);

- Keeping cold water in the fridge at all times. Buy a water pitcher or a water filtering jug and place it at the front of your fridge. It needs to be visible and easy to reach to be convenient;

- Knowing your environment. Do a tour of your workplace to remind yourself of where the water fountains or coolers are. Check if the cafeteria charges for hot water or if there's a vending machine that sells water bottles close by;

- Buy a smaller water bottle to carry in your purse or backpack for when you're on the go. Ideally, it should hold no more than one to two cups. Large water bottles are often intimidating and if they are too heavy or bulky, they're more likely to get left behind;

- Leave a reusable water bottle in your car at all times so that you always have some on-hand.

Get excited and add some flavour by...

- Trying infused water. Add one of the following combinations to your water pitcher or water bottle:

  ✓ Sliced cucumber + fresh mint leaves;
  ✓ Sliced strawberries + fresh basil leaves;
  ✓ Sliced lemon + fresh lavender;
  ✓ Blackberries + fresh thyme;
  ✓ One cinnamon stick (for best results leave overnight in your water bottle);

- Using flavoured ice cubes. This idea involves freezing concentrated fruit purees, spirals of citrus rinds, and/or fresh herbs into ice cube trays. Adding one to three of these ice cubes into your water not only adds a fun flavour and keeps your water colder, but it's also a colourful touch. This is a great alternative to store-bought water enhancers that contain artificial sweeteners.

- E.g. puree two cups of chopped watermelon with the juice of one lime. Freeze the mixture in ice cube trays. Add two ice cubes into your reusable water bottle;

- Making a homemade tea with an added twist. Add eight ounces (one cup) of boiling water to the combinations below. Drink hot or refrigerate overnight and enjoy cold.

  - ✓ 1/2 sliced lemon + 1/2 inch piece of peeled fresh ginger + 1 tsp honey;
  - ✓ A green tea bag + fresh mint leaves;
  - ✓ A black tea bag + orange slices or peach slices;
  - ✓ A earl grey tea bag + sprig of lavender + lemon slices + 1 tsp honey;
  - ✓ A white tea bag + mint leaves + dash of lime juice;

- Treating yourself to some loose tea leaves or flavoured tea bags at specialty shops.

Set reminders by…

- Downloading an app. There are countless free apps out there to help you track your daily water intake and even ones that will send you constant reminders throughout the day to drink;

- Add a sticky note to your computer monitor. Be sure to change the placement of the sticky note every week so it doesn't blend into the background;

- If you're someone who does repetitive tasks at work, use this to your advantage! For example, challenge yourself to take three sips of water every time you read a new email and every time you send an email;

- Buy a 'time stamped' water bottle or simply recreate one by writing the hours of your work day down the side of your bottle with a permanent marker. For example, evenly space 9 a.m., 10 a.m., 11 a.m., and 12 a.m. down one side of the bottle and 1 p.m., 2 p.m., 3 p.m., and 4 p.m. down the opposite side of the bottle. This strategy will also help you to pace yourself throughout the day.

CHAPTER 5:

Protein

Why is protein so important?

Protein is something we spend *a lot* of time talking about with our patients before and after surgery. Whether you're a meat lover, vegetarian, or vegan, eating enough protein is key to short and long term success after WLS for a number of reasons:

- You heal better, and faster, after surgery;
- Protein helps maintain your muscles while you're losing weight;
- It keeps cravings in check since protein helps you feel fuller longer (i.e. eating just an apple may keep you full for 15 to 30 minutes, but if you add a protein alongside it, like ¼ cup nuts, 100 g Greek yogurt, or 50 g of cheese, you'll feel full for 2-3 hours);
- To prevent hair loss;
- To avoid low energy and fatigue.

How much protein do I need?

This is a great question for your WLS dietitian because everyone's needs are different. Your WLS dietitian will take into account the following when calculating your daily protein needs:

- Your height, weight, and body composition (i.e. do you have a lot of muscle?);
- Which surgery you had;
- How active you are (i.e. do you have a physical job? How often and how intensely you workout?, etc.);
- How well your hunger is controlled;
- Your medical conditions (i.e. do you have kidney disease?).

To give you a general idea of what your protein needs are use the following calculation (NOTE: this calculation assumes you're healthy):

- Lap band, sleeve gastrectomy, and gastric bypass = 1.1 g/kg of your IBW (ideal body weight)
- Duodenal switch = 1.5 g/kg of your IBW (ideal body weight)

These estimations are simply that, an estimation. Speak with your WLS dietitian for a more specific and personalized number.

The top five foods that people mistake for being high in protein

1. Hummus

The average store-bought hummus has just one gram of protein per tablespoon. Homemade hummus, however, is typically slightly higher in protein. Instead, opt for homemade hummus, homemade black bean dip or homemade tzatziki (made with Greek yogurt) as dips for your veggies. All of these dips are significantly higher in protein when made at home compared to their store-bought counterparts.

2. Cream cheese

The average cream cheese has only one gram of protein per tablespoon. You're better off choosing ricotta cheese or a nut butter instead. Instead, opt for ricotta cheese (with a sprinkle of sunflower seeds and a drizzle of honey!) or peanut butter on your morning toast.

3. Chicken broth

The average store bought chicken broth has only one gram of protein per cup. For this reason, your WLS team will likely recommended you choose higher protein soups immediately after surgery (e.g. milk based soups and pureed legume soups). Instead, opt for more filling thicker soups, such as a curried lentil soup, a roasted red pepper black bean soup, or a hearty chili.

4. Quinoa

Quinoa is a filling grain product not because of its protein content, but because of its fibre. While it's the only grain listed as a 'complete' protein, it only has two grams of protein per ¼ cup of cooked quinoa. Make sure to always top your quinoa with meat, fish, legumes, or tofu to meet your daily protein needs.

5. Almond, cashew, and rice milks

These alternative milks contain a measly one gram of protein per cup. Cow's milk and soy milk are much better alternatives if you're looking for a good source of protein.

When is a protein shake or bar a good idea?

Although protein shakes and bars aren't always necessary, there *are* times that including them in your menu is a good idea.

When you're not able to meet your protein needs with food alone. Protein shakes and bars are best used when you know that you're not getting enough protein from the food you eat. For example, you may be eating three meals and two to three snacks every day, but in the first few months after surgery—because your portions are still small—you may not meet your estimated protein needs. If your WLS dietitian is telling you that you're eating well, choosing the right foods, and eating often enough, but you're still not getting enough protein then a daily protein shake or bar is definitely a good idea.

When you're too busy to have a meal or snack. Grabbing a protein shake or bar is always a better option than skipping a meal or snack. Whether you're too busy at work to take a pause for lunch or your errands took longer than you anticipated, a protein shake or bar is an easy meal replacement. Ideally, this should not be a daily habit. If you're starting to notice that you seem to be too busy for meals and snacks on a regular basis it's a good idea to meet with your WLS dietitian to discuss other quick and convenient foods options that are more balanced.

When you're not hungry or don't feel like eating, but it's time to eat. Again, having a protein shake is better than skipping a meal and liquid meals tend to go down easier when you don't have an appetite.

After exercise. A protein shake or bar is also a good idea to have after exercising if you know that you won't be eating a meal or snack within an hour. If you spent the past hour weight training, interval training, or endurance training, it's important to choose a supplement that contains 15 g protein and 15-30 g carbohydrates. One cup of milk mixed with 4 tablespoons of Greek yogurt or ¼ cup of silken tofu would have the carbohydrates and protein needed. Alternatively, a 15 g protein shake with one fruit (or ½ cup of fruit) blended together would work too.

When is a protein shake or bar not a good idea?

The answer to this question depends on *why* you are reaching for the protein shake or bar. What is the motivation behind your decision to choose a protein supplement over real food?

First off, it's important to know that protein shakes and bars aren't better than eating real food. Protein supplements are often missing carbohydrates, fibre, and good fats, which are all important parts of a healthy diet. Keep in mind that WLS isn't the quick dieting fix that you may have been after, before undergoing the surgery. You won't realistically be able to replace your meals with protein shakes and bars your whole life.

If you are relying on protein shakes or bars more often than one to two times a week, it is important to choose options that are more balanced. Look for protein shakes with 20 g of protein which also contain 15-30 g of carbohydrates. Otherwise, if there's less than 5 g of carbohydrates per serving, blend half a banana or ½ cup of fruit into your shake.

Ultimately, if a shake is meant to increase your protein and is added to your day, that's fine. But if the shake is meant to replace meals several times a week, it's important that you include carbohydrates in that shake.

Using a protein shake or bar to cleanse, reset, or mimic the liquid diet you were on before surgery in order to lose weight faster, is not appropriate after surgery.

How do I choose the right protein powders, protein shakes, and protein bars?

The protein supplement industry is huge and can be difficult to navigate. It's important to focus on the nutrition facts tables and ingredient lists of supplements. Ignore the front of package labels as they can often be misleading when selecting a product.

Protein powder
Protein powders are meant to be mixed with water or milk prior to drinking. They can be convenient if you don't want to bring heavy, ready-to-drink shakes around with you.

When looking for protein powders, the first ingredient should be 'whey protein isolate or concentrate,' or 'soy protein isolate or concentrate.' These types of protein are 'complete proteins,' meaning that your body will absorb most of the protein listed in the nutrition facts table and they provide all 9 essential amino acids (i.e. the building blocks of protein). You may find other products that use 'rice protein' or 'pea protein,' and while these may be easier to digest, they're not complete proteins. This means that your body will absorb a smaller amount of the protein indicated on the label and that they're missing many of the essential amino acids your body needs (i.e. amino acids that your body can't produce by itself, and that need to come from your food).

When looking at the nutrition facts table of a protein powder, be sure to keep an eye out for a few things:

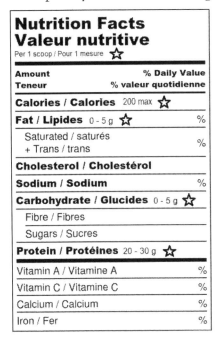

- Look at the suggested portion at the top of the nutrition facts table;
- There should be between 20 to 30 g of protein per portion;
- There should be between 0 to 5 g of carbohydrates per portion;
- There should be between 0 to 5 g of fat per portion;
- Most flavoured whey and soy protein supplements use artificial sweeteners. If you wish to avoid these, choose the unflavoured options and add your own blended fruit, vanilla extract, or cocoa powder to your protein shakes.

Ready-to-drink protein shakes

There is also the option of ready-to-drink protein shakes. No preparation necessary, just open and start sipping. These shakes are convenient when you have little time or no equipment on hand to measure your protein powder, add water, and blend.

Like other shakes, ready-to-drink protein shakes should have 'whey protein isolate or concentrate,' or 'soy protein isolate or concentrate' as the first ingredient so you absorb the most protein and get the amino acids your body needs.

When looking at the nutrition facts table of a protein shake, be sure to keep an eye out for a few things:

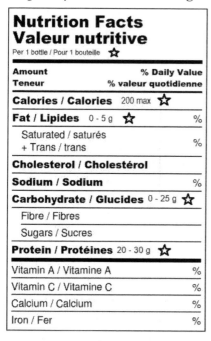

- Look at the suggested portion at the top of the nutrition facts table;
- There should be between 20 to 30 g of protein per portion;
- There should be between 0 to 25 g of carbohydrates per portion;
- There should be between 0 to 5 g of fat per portion;
- Ready-to-drink protein shakes can be sweetened with artificial sweeteners or sugar. The one you choose comes down to personal

preference, however it's important to remember that if you've had a gastric bypass, you're at risk of experiencing dumping syndrome if the carbohydrates (or sugar content) is too high. This will occur if the sugar is coming from added sugars, but might not occur if the sugars are more natural (like those coming from unsweetened milk).

Protein bars

Protein bars are a convenient, lightweight option that you can keep in a purse or in your pocket. They store well in office desks, gym bags, and even in your car. This option will only work if you're already eating solid foods and are not experiencing any digestive issues, otherwise the texture may be too difficult or will feel too heavy. In this case, a protein shake or powder may be a better solution for you. Most bars include some poor quality fats (including trans fats) which have been linked to heart disease.

Like all protein supplements, the first ingredient should be complete proteins like 'whey protein isolate or concentrate,' or 'soy protein isolate or concentrate.' You might find some bars that say they include a 'protein blend', but we suggest you look for the previously mentioned proteins instead.

When looking at the nutrition facts table of a protein bar, be sure to keep an eye out for a few things:

Nutrition Facts
Valeur nutritive
Per 1 bar / Pour 1 barre ☆

Amount Teneur	% Daily Value % valeur quotidienne
Calories / Calories 300 max ☆	
Fat / Lipides 0 - 5 g ☆	%
Saturated / saturés + Trans / trans	%
Cholesterol / Cholestérol	
Sodium / Sodium	%
Carbohydrate / Glucides 0 - 25 g ☆	
Fibre / Fibres 3 g or more / ou plus ☆	
Sugars / Sucres 0 - 10 g ☆	
Protein / Protéines 20 - 30 g ☆	
Vitamin A / Vitamine A	%
Vitamin C / Vitamine C	%
Calcium / Calcium	%
Iron / Fer	%

- Look at the suggested portion at the top of the nutrition facts table. While this usually states a portion is the whole bar, some may indicate the nutrition facts are for only half of it;
- There should be between 20 to 30 g of protein per portion;
- There should be between 0 to 25 g of carbohydrates per portion;
- There should be 10 g or less of sugar per portion;
- There should be between 0 to 5 g of fat per portion;
- There should be as close to 0 g of trans fats as possible;
- Try to look for a protein bar that includes some fibre (ideally there should be a minimum of 3g of fibre per bar). This may be harder to find, but it's worth it to keep a healthy digestive tract;
- Some protein bars use sugar while others use artificial sweeteners, so be sure to choose the right one for you.

CHAPTER 6:

Delaying Fluids

Why can't I eat and drink at the same time?

Not drinking and eating at the same time is not only one of the biggest changes in terms of eating habits with surgery, but it's also one of the most important new habits. From our experience, patients who eat and drink at the same time lose less weight in the first year after surgery, and are more likely to regain weight in the years following WLS.

Why?

Basically, whatever liquid you have during your meal or snack, helps flush the food out of your stomach and into your intestines. As a result, you feel less full at meals and are hungry soon after eating. By delaying your fluids (i.e. waiting at least 30 minutes after eating to start drinking again) you allow the food to stay in your stomach longer, which causes you to feel full earlier and more satisfied with smaller portions.

Take a moment to think of this (unfortunate) analogy:

Eating food to fill up your stomach is like filling up a toilet bowl. Taking sips of liquid during or right after eating is like flushing, with the water taking everything away and leaving the bowl empty. The same happens when you drink, as it quickly empties the food from your stomach.

Essentially, eating and drinking at the same time is a way of cheating the surgery.

Consequences of drinking while eating, or drinking soon after, include:

- Being able to consume portions that are larger than usual (i.e. more than one cup);
- Never feeling full nor satisfied when eating;
- Feeling true hunger soon after eating;
- Being more likely to nibble on food between meals and snacks.

Delaying your fluids is especially important for those of you who have had the gastric bypass.

Why?

Because you no longer have a pyloric sphincter (the valve that connects your stomach to your intestines). In a normal stomach, this valve helps regulate and control the flow of our food. After surgery, and without this valve, your digestive system becomes more like a waterslide. Liquid entering your stomach will flush all the food into your intestines without any resistance.

How long should I be waiting between eating and drinking?

It's recommended you wait at least 30 minutes after you've finished eating before drinking. It's also advised to stop drinking 15 minutes before you eat. Although this habit is difficult to get used to in the beginning, it gets easier with time. Before you know it, it'll be your new normal.

If you've already had surgery and are still eating and drinking at the same time, we urge you to start working on this ASAP! The further out you are from surgery, the harder it is to get back on track. Although it'll take time (likely months) to start seeing small increases in your portion sizes or notice an increased frequency of eating, these subtle changes will start creeping up on you, followed by a gradual weight regain.

Tips:

- Don't keep your glass, mug, or water bottle on the table while you're eating as it'll make drinking *way* less tempting (out of sight, out of mind);

- Make sure you're sipping on water up until 15 minutes before your meal or snack so you're less likely to be thirsty when eating;

- Download an app like 'Bariatric Timer' (it's free!) to help you keep track of time between drinking and meals;

- If you have a smart watch, set a timer to keep track of time more discreetly.

Why am I told to avoid soup after surgery?

There are two main reasons that soups are discouraged after surgery:

1. Soup is both liquid and solid. Soup is the meal equivalent of eating and drinking at the same time.

2. Soups are typically low in protein and therefore less filling. Often our patients will choose chicken noodle soup because

they find it comforting. But with only four tiny cubes of chicken floating around in their bowl, it's not enough protein to keep them full nor meet their protein needs.

Does this mean I can never have soup again?

Absolutely not. Having soup once in a while is fine. We just discourage patients from having it on a daily, or even weekly, basis.

To make soup a healthier, more WLS friendly choice, there are a few things you can do:

- If the soup is a side dish, eat only the solid pieces in your soup (i.e. vegetables, meat, legumes, etc.) and leave the broth behind. Otherwise, wait 15 to 30 minutes after finishing the soup to eat the main meal;

- If the soup is your main meal, then choose protein-rich soups like cream-style soups (prepared with milk) or a thick lentil soup, split pea soup, chili, or stew-style soups that contain a good serving of meat, poultry, fish, or beans;

- An ideal soup is broken down into ½ cup of protein rich foods, ½ cup of cooked vegetables, and a couple tablespoons of broth. If you can easily count the number of beans or pieces of meat in your bowl, then there definitely isn't enough protein. Either add in more meat/beans, or add one ounce of cheese on the side of your meal;

- If you're purchasing canned soups or chili, try to choose soups that have close to 10-15 g of protein per one-cup serving (this can be really difficult to find);

- The true test of whether your soup is a good choice, is how long it keeps you full. If you're truly hungry (stomach hunger, not head hunger) within one to two hours after your soup, it wasn't a good choice. Ideally, you should feel satisfied for two to three hours after eating.

The bottom line: Soup is often very satisfying in the first couple of months after surgery, but longer term, and especially if it's lacking in protein, it will no longer be enough.

Does this mean I need to avoid cereal too?

Cereal is similar to soup: solids mixed with liquid. However, like soups, there are some cereals which are higher in protein than others. Choose cereals that have at least 5 g of protein per half cup (before adding milk).

One cup of cereal may fill you up in the first six months after surgery, but as you approach your anniversary, you may notice that you need a larger and larger portion to feel satisfied. Once you begin to notice this, it's recommended that you opt for a solid breakfast instead. Or simply serve your cereal over 1/3 cup of Greek yogurt instead of adding milk.

CHAPTER 7:
Dumping Syndrome

What is dumping syndrome?

Dumping syndrome is a reaction that occurs most commonly after having had a gastric bypass when you eat too much sugar at once. Trigger foods include: large portions of ice cream, juice, milkshakes, candy, chocolate, pie, rich desserts, etc.

After a gastric bypass your body no longer has the valve (also known as the pyloric sphincter) between the stomach and the intestines. The job of the pyloric sphincter is to keep food in the stomach until it's ready to be absorbed in your intestines. With the gastric bypass, you no longer have this helpful valve, so undigested food and concentrated sugars enter the small intestine easily and quickly. This causes a variety of uncomfortable symptoms.

There are two types of dumping syndrome, early and late.

Early dumping syndrome
In early dumping syndrome, symptoms are felt within 15-30 minutes after eating a concentrated amount of sugar. Symptoms include sweating, light-headedness, nausea, bloating, cramping, diarrhea, and a fast heart rate.

Why does this happen?

The small intestine dislikes the undigested concentrated sugars, so it responds by pulling water from your bloodstream into your intestines to dilute and flush out the sugar. This rush of excess fluid in your intestines results in diarrhea, a classic sign of dumping syndrome.

Late dumping syndrome

In late dumping syndrome, symptoms are felt within one to three hours after eating a concentrated amount of sugar. Symptoms include weakness, sweating, shakiness, reduced concentration, and dizziness. The experience is similar to that of a low blood sugar episode, or a hypoglycemic reaction.

While dumping syndrome is commonly associated with a gastric bypass, there have been a few stories of patients with the sleeve gastrectomy who've experienced dumping syndrome when eating large amount of sweets. Although this is uncommon, it may still occur.

Which foods cause dumping syndrome?

The good news is that dumping syndrome can be prevented. Dumping syndrome happens after eating a large amount of concentrated sugars (i.e. foods that are high in sugar). Concentrated sugars are found most often in highly processed foods like milkshakes, ice cream, cakes, cookies, muffins, chocolate bars, sugar-sweetened beverages, fruit juice (even the no-sugar added kind), and sugary cereals.

It's very uncommon that dumping syndrome will happen after eating fresh fruit, bread, rice, and potatoes (i.e. foods containing complex and simple carbohydrates), but there are always a few exceptions. For example, a homemade smoothie loaded with pineapple juice and mangoes has been a trigger for a couple of our patients in the past.

Does this mean I can never eat sweets again?

Most patients who've had a gastric bypass will say they can have a small portion of dessert, but are unable to eat the same larger portions that they ate before surgery. At the end of the day, it all comes down to the amount of sugar in a specific food, meaning, if a particular dessert has less sugar than another, you may be able to eat a few more bites of it.

Everyone has a different limit as to how much sugar they can tolerate. If the treat you're eating has a nutrition facts table, use this to give yourself an idea of the portion size that you can likely tolerate safely. A safe portion is one with 20-30 g or less of carbohydrates and 10-15 g or less of sugar. This would typically mean one to two cookies, ⅓ - ½ cup of ice cream, or less than half of a chocolate bar. These small amounts mean you can occasionally treat yourself, however, you are limited to tasting rather than indulging.

Another tip is to look at the ingredient list. If glucose, fructose, sucrose, cane sugar, and syrups are within the first three ingredients, this food product is likely too high in simple sugars for your new stomach.

What do I do if I'm in the middle of a reaction?

If you're experiencing early dumping syndrome, there is little that can be done to treat this. You'll have to wait it out and be more careful next time.

If you're experiencing late dumping syndrome (i.e. hypoglycemic reaction, or low blood sugar reaction) you can take the following steps:

Step one:
Test your blood sugar if you have a glucometer (a meter that tests your blood sugar). If your blood sugar is less than four (4.0 mmol/L) move on to step two. If you don't have a glucometer to test your blood sugar, but you're feeling symptoms of low blood sugar (i.e. weakness, sweating, shakiness, reduced concentration, and dizziness), you should also move on to step two.

Step two:
Quickly have one of the following:

- ½ cup of juice (not diet juice);
- 1 tablespoon of honey;
- 1 tablespoon of maple syrup;
- 3-4 dextrose tablets (you can find these in any pharmacy).

Step three:
Sit down and relax for 15 minutes. If you have a glucometer test your blood sugar once more after 15 minutes to be sure your level is now above four (4.0 mmol/L). If you don't have a glucometer and the symptoms have not reduced, or if your blood sugar is still less than four, repeat step two again.

Step four:
Now that your blood sugar is no longer low, you'll need to keep your blood sugar level stable. If your next meal or snack is more than one hour away, immediately have one portion of protein (e.g. 30 g cheese, ¼ cup nuts, or 2 tablespoons of peanut butter).

You may be worried about step two, which is advising you to have some sugar. If eating sugar caused this problem in the first place, why would we advise you to have MORE sugar? Because when your blood sugar is low, the only way to bring it up quickly is to have sugar. The amount of sugar that is recommended to treat your low blood sugar, is likely a lesser amount than what caused your dumping syndrome. The sugar will increase your blood sugar and the protein will keep it there. If you miss the protein snack, within the hour, you risk having another episode of dumping syndrome.

Treating an episode is a necessary step, however this isn't a trick or a solution that should encourage you to eat more sweets. If you've experienced dumping syndrome, the best treatment is to avoid sweets altogether or limit your intake to one to two bites rather than indulging.

NOTE: If you're driving and you start to feel the symptoms mentioned above, pull your car over immediately. It's dangerous to drive while experiencing a low blood sugar reaction.

CHAPTER 8:
Hair Loss

Why am I losing my hair?

Hair shedding is unfortunately an unpleasant side effect of WLS, mostly attributed to rapid weight loss. This phenomenon is also called 'shock loss' or telogen effluvium. Hair shedding is basically a response to the emotional and physiological stress that your body undergoes in the months after surgery.

Hair shedding is normal after surgery up until around eight to ten months. As your weight begins to stabilize (usually around eight to twelve months after surgery), your hair will start to grow back. Before you freak out—because we know you are!—we want to reassure you that hair shedding doesn't happen to the majority of patients (less than half of patients) and if you are one of the patients who does experience it, we promise you won't go completely bald. Your hair will simply look thinner for a little while.

NOTE: If you're still experiencing significant hair loss after 12 months, you should contact your WLS team immediately. This isn't normal and likely indicates an underlying micronutrient deficiency.

Is there anything I can do to prevent hair loss?

Unfortunately, there is nothing that you can do that will 100% prevent hair loss, but there are 4 things that you can do to help prevent *excessive* hair shedding.

1. Meet your protein needs.
Firstly, it's super important to meet your protein needs. Speak with your WLS dietitian to know how many grams of protein you should be consuming every day.

2. Take your vitamins.
Secondly, it's crucial that you take your prescribed vitamins every day. It's also important to make sure that the vitamins you're taking have been approved by your WLS team. There are many incomplete vitamins on the market, including gummy multivitamins, so make sure you're taking the right ones.

3. Eat a well-balanced diet.
Thirdly, consuming enough calories and having a well-balanced diet is key. Malnutrition is a common cause of hair loss. Although the goal of WLS is for you to be consuming less calories, there *is* such a thing as too few calories.

4. Don't skip your blood tests!
Lastly, we want to stress that having regular blood tests—as suggested by your WLS team—especially within the first year after surgery are key to screening for nutritional deficiencies (such as iron, zinc, and copper) that can worsen hair loss.

Many patients ask us about using nutritional supplements such as biotin, omega-3s, hair, skin and nail supplements, and special shampoos or serums, however none of these products will significantly prevent hair loss after WLS.

CHAPTER 9:
Alcohol

How will I react to alcohol after surgery?

After WLS, especially after a gastric bypass, alcohol is absorbed quickly into the bloodstream. This means that you'll feel the effects of alcohol much faster on a much smaller portion of alcohol than you would have before surgery. This happens for two reasons:

1. You have less of the enzyme in the stomach that helps your body digest alcohol, meaning you'll feel the effects quickly;

2. You're losing weight! You reach a higher blood alcohol level faster at a lower weight.

Just as you'll feel the effects of alcohol more quickly, it'll also take longer for the alcohol to leave your system. For this reason, we strongly encourage you to test your new tolerance slowly, and do so at home. We also recommend that you start with small sips as opposed to full drinks. Pour ⅓ to ½ of the portion you would normally pour yourself.

NOTE: It's important to know that even one standard alcoholic drink in some patients can be enough to raise their blood alcohol concentration above the legal driving limit. Research says that on average, the effects of alcohol can be four to six times more intense in gastric bypass patients. This means one portion of wine (five ounces) has the potential to hit you like four to six glasses of wine.

For this reason, we strongly encourage you to abstain from alcohol completely if you're planning on driving anywhere that same night.

When can I start drinking again after surgery?

It's typically recommended to avoid alcohol for the first six months after surgery. After this point it may be safe to have the occasional drink, but research shows that the less you drink after surgery, the better your chances are of keeping the weight off.

Alcohol is also a stomach irritant, and drinking it soon after surgery may increase your risk of developing stomach ulcers.

If you do decide to drink socially, there are a few tips you can use to make better choices while out with friends:

- Pour yourself half servings to account for your new tolerance;
- Add ice cubes or water to mixed drinks to dilute the alcohol content;
- Pace yourself;
- Have water between alcoholic beverages;
- Limit social drinking to a maximum of two alcoholic drinks, or less, in an evening;
- To avoid the stigma of not drinking, have a beverage of your choice in a wine glass (add a splash of cranberry juice or low calorie water flavouring to your water to mimic the colour of a rosé, and no one will know the difference!);
- Take a taxi home or have a designated driver before the evening begins.

What type of alcohol is best for me now?

Alcohol is a source of liquid calories with no nutritive value. We're often asked which type of alcohol is best after surgery. Unfortunately, there's no right answer to this, but it's important to consider a few factors:

- Beer, sparkling wine, and champagne are carbonated beverages which should be avoided after surgery;
- Mixed drinks that contain juice may have a high enough sugar content to trigger dumping syndrome if you have a gastric bypass;
- Alcohol is a liquid and liquids should not be consumed while eating;
- Alcohol on an empty stomach can irritate your stomach and intestines, and so smaller portions are recommended.

Although general alcohol guidelines suggest limiting alcohol to ten drinks a week for women and 15 drinks a week for men, studies have shown that after WLS these amounts can lead to weight regain in the long term. Those who drank less than two drinks a week were more likely to keep the weight off, and those who drank nine drinks a week or more were the ones who regained weight five years after their gastric bypass. Although this study didn't look into other types of WLS, it's likely that similar results would be seen among patients with the sleeve gastrectomy or duodenal switch due to the extra calories.

Alcohol abuse

Unfortunately, there are higher levels of alcohol abuse among patients who've had WLS as compared to people who haven't. It's thought that this may be due to a transfer of addiction. When someone depends on food to cope with their stress and emotions, and they can no longer eat a large enough amount of food to soothe them, sometimes they turn to alcohol to cope after surgery since it takes very little to feel its effects.

There is also some research that suggests that alcohol is more addictive after gastric bypass surgery because of how quick and intense the effects are (i.e. similar to that of addictive drugs).

We encourage you to reach out to your WLS team if you feel that your new alcohol habits are becoming a concern, or if you no longer feel in control.

CHAPTER 10:

Caffeine

How much coffee can I have after surgery?

The truth is, we don't have enough research to suggest that caffeine needs to be completely avoided, however it *is* suggested to follow the general guidelines which encourage caffeine be limited and consumed in moderation.

Surgery or no surgery, studies show that we should be limiting our intake of coffee to 400 mg/day, or three to four cups of coffee a day (depending on the brew) in healthy adults. Drinking more than this can cause stomach upset, sleeplessness, restlessness, and irritability.

It used to be thought that caffeine was a diuretic, causing your body to lose more water than you're drinking. However, over the years it's been shown that this doesn't seem to be the case. While caffeine *can* dehydrate you, it does so minimally, especially with a moderate intake (i.e. less than four true cups [250 ml cups]). For this reason we count coffee in your fluid intake up to three to four cups. Keep in mind that this may not be the case with higher caffeine intakes (i.e. five or more cups a day).

There are some additional reasons you should consider limiting your caffeine intake further:

Reflux or heartburn

If you've had the sleeve gastrectomy or the duodenal switch procedures, you have a higher risk of having reflux or heartburn problems. While medication can help reduce these symptoms, it's important to cut out the problem rather than treat the symptoms. Cut the amount of coffee you're drinking in half or switch to decaf to see if your caffeine habits are part of the problem.

Symptoms

If you experience an upset stomach, sleeplessness, irritability or restlessness, you may want to consider reducing your caffeine intake for a few weeks to see if these symptoms resolve. To improve your quality of sleep, it's recommended to avoid caffeine products after 2:00 p.m.

Calories

Coffee and tea, with nothing else added, contain zero calories. The moment we start adding sugar, milk, cream, and coffee whitener, the calories begin to add up.

The bottom line: Despite not having enough research to give you a definitive final answer, it's suggested you limit caffeine to low or moderate amounts (i.e. less than three to four cups a day) especially in the first month after surgery, when your stomach is most sensitive after surgery. Choose decaf coffee or herbal tea more often, and use a smaller coffee mug to help reduce your intake.

Tip: It's difficult to drink enough water after surgery. For this reason, a good after surgery goal is to wait until you can drink at least one litre of water a day before introducing caffeinated beverages.

NOTE: Caffeine pills are also discouraged. If you're having issues with fatigue, speak with your WLS dietitian or WLS team. Fatigue is often a sign of dehydration and poor eating habits.

CHAPTER 11:

Calories & Carbs

How many calories do I need per day?

This is the most common question that patients ask us. For several reasons, our answer isn't what patients want nor expect to hear.

Answer:
We don't give out daily calorie limits or ranges, because we honestly don't know what they are!

There's currently a lot of debate on what patients' calorie needs are after WLS. The equations traditionally used to estimate how many calories a non-WLS patient needs per day don't seem to be accurate after WLS.

What do we recommend?
Instead of counting calories, we encourage patients to focus on meeting their protein needs, distributing this protein appropriately throughout the day and balancing out their meals and snacks with fruits, vegetables, and grain products. Limiting your total portions at meals to around one cup naturally limits your calorie intake.

Listening to your body's cues is key to help limit portion sizes and, as a result, also helps limit your calorie intake. If you're listening to your body's hunger and satiety cues, you're likely on track in terms of daily calories*.

Listen to your body. It's the most accurate calorie counter that you have, and more importantly, it's tailored to you better than any equations will ever be!

*Although this is not accurate in the months after surgery when you are experiencing little to no hunger cues! In the months after surgery, it's recommended to follow the meal and snack portions recommended by your WLS dietitian and to stop eating before you feel nauseous or uncomfortable.

Does this mean I shouldn't look at the calories on products?

You should still look at the nutrition facts tables on the foods you buy so you can compare products and make educated choices. However, we want to remind you that a food can't be determined healthy or unhealthy just by looking at its calorie content. You need to look at the other numbers on the panel too, so take a step back and look at what type of food you're holding, and use common sense.

For example, if you compare instant oatmeal and oatmeal cookies for breakfast, you might find them to be fairly comparable in calories (if you only eat what the label says is one portion). However, if you continue reading the nutrition fact table you'll find that oatmeal (made with milk) has more protein and fibre than the cookies, meaning you'll feel fuller longer. Oatmeal also has a bunch of vitamins and minerals that are useful to your body and it contains significantly less sugar. The lesson is to never judge foods based solely on calories.

Let's look at another example:

A portion of nuts (¼ cup) is significantly higher in calories than a portion of rice crackers. Many of our patients are scared off from the calorie content of nuts and seeds, and may instead choose the rice crackers as a snack option. This is an example of when you need to use common sense and take a step back to look at what each food is offering you, and what it will do for your body.

Nuts contain healthy fats, protein, fibre, and minerals that nourish your body. Yes the calories from their fats and protein add up quickly, but they are what keep you full. Rice crackers, on the other hand, contain only a small amount of carbohydrates, lots of air, and little to no nutritional value. Great snack? Not quite. While it's not a bad option when accompanied with peanut butter or cheese (both of which are protein sources), the rice crackers alone will not keep you feeling satisfied for very long. You will likely find yourself looking for something else to eat fifteen minutes later.

Moral of the story: Calories are not the enemy!

I heard I should be avoiding carbohydrates, is this true?

This is 100% false! Carbohydrates are the body's preferred source of fuel. Just as your car needs gas to run, your body and brain rely on carbohydrates to give you the physical and mental energy that you need to get through your day.

What are carbohydrates actually?

The majority of patients identify carbohydrates simply as grain products (e.g. bread, pasta, and rice). When dieters say they're going on a low carb diet, they typically plan to eliminate or reduce their consumption of these grain products.

In reality, carbohydrate sources include many other foods, like milk, yogurt, fruit, plenty of vegetables, and legumes.

Did you know that one cup of milk has the same amount of grams of carbohydrates as a piece of toast? Or that a large apple has twice as many grams of carbohydrates as that same slice of toast? Or that a ½ cup of chickpeas has three times the amount of carbohydrates as the toast?

Confused?

This is why we challenge our patients in *why* they want to experiment with low-carbohydrate diets. *What* does that mean to them? And *which* foods are they planning on restricting? A lower carbohydrate diet is not necessarily a healthier one!

In a world where our food apps can track everything, it's sometimes hard to make sense of all of the numbers they give us. You shouldn't be blindly trying to decrease your total grams of carbohydrates or total grams of fat per day without understanding how that translates into food choices and your overall health.

The *type* of carbohydrate is more important than the *amount* of carbohydrate.

Not all carbohydrates are created equal.

The most common forms of carbohydrates are:

- **Fibre** (for the purposes of this book, we will refer to fibre as a 'complex carbohydrates');

- **Sugar** (for the purposes of this book, we will refer to them as 'simple carbohydrates').
- **Starch**. Starch is calculated by taking the total carbohydrates and subtracting both the fibre and sugar from it (for the purposes of this book, we will refer to starches as 'complex carbohydrates').

Foods that are high in carbohydrates but contain a fair amount of fibre and starch, and a low amount of sugar (i.e. high in complex carbohydrates and low in simple carbohydrates), are typically healthier choices. Complex carbohydrates take longer to digest, which is why they make you feel fuller longer.

Examples include:

- Barley;
- Oats;
- Quinoa;
- Whole-grain products;
- Legumes.

Similarly, foods that are high in carbohydrates but contain high amounts of sugar and low amounts of fibre and starch (i.e. high in simple carbohydrates and low in complex carbohydrates) are typically less healthy choices. Simple carbohydrates are quickly digested, which is why they give you a quick boost of energy, but also why you don't feel satisfied for very long.

Examples include:

- Pastries;
- Donuts;
- Chocolate;

- Candy;
- Juice;
- Regular soda;
- Sugary cereals.

After WLS, protein should always be eaten first, followed by your vegetables and then your grain products (e.g. rice, quinoa, pasta) or starch (e.g. potato, sweet potato, squash). Eating in this order will naturally limit the amount of carbohydrates you consume at each meal because of the limited space in your stomach.

Patients who restrict their carbohydrate intake, in our experience, typically have a harder time finding a healthy balance and joy in eating again. One of the biggest consequences of skipping out on carbohydrates at mealtime is that your blood sugar is less balanced, which can result in sugar cravings later on in the day.

Remember: All foods fit, but it's the portions of food that should be the focus in a healthy diet, post WLS.

CHAPTER 12:

Portions & Structure

How often should I be eating?

You should aim to have three meals and two to three snacks in your day.

All WLS centres will agree that all patients should have three meals every day. These shouldn't be skipped and should become routine. Skipping meals leads to grazing later on in the day, and in the long term could lead you back to old bad habits. When it comes to snacks, most centres will suggest two to three snacks per day. Having snacks helps you to get all the protein you need in your day, which is difficult—even impossible—to get with just three meals. Research also shows that patients who were the most successful at losing weight after surgery were those who ate two to three snacks daily.

Having snacks is an organized activity. You have to plan them ahead of time. Snacking can help prevent grazing (or mindlessly picking at food), which is unplanned, not measured, and often driven by emotion. Grazing leads us to eat large amounts of food over an extended period of time, like eating a whole bag of popcorn or chips while watching several episodes of our favourite show. We don't plan for it to happen, it just does.

Having regular snacks helps reduce cravings by keeping you satisfied and in control, which ultimately keeps your eating habits more structured. Ideally, your snacks should be distributed throughout the day, one between breakfast and lunch, another between lunch and dinner, and perhaps another after supper. Studies show that keeping most of your calories for the evening, even if you're not overeating, can lead to weight gain in the average person.

If you find yourself having two snacks after dinner, you might not be eating enough during the day. Being organized is key. Planning your snacks ahead of time (e.g. an apple with a handful of nuts, or a protein bar) and storing them in convenient places can help keep you on track throughout the day.

Why should I weigh and measure my food?

It's really important to weigh and measure all of your food on a regular basis. Initially your stomach will be a good guide to manage your portions. But you'll begin to notice that by three months after surgery you can eat more than you did five weeks out. By six months you're eating more than at three months, and at one year you're eating more than at six months!

For this reason, we strongly suggest that you weigh and measure your food throughout your WLS journey.

That being said, we've never met anyone who weighs and measures their food every day for their entire life. It's not a realistic, nor a healthy habit to have. But we do suggest that you weigh and measure your food every day for the first two to three months, and then only once or twice a month after this point. This will help keep you in check to verify if, and by how much, your portions have increased. Over time you'll be able to approximate the amount you can eat by using the same sized plates, the same sized cups, same bowls, and containers. This will help you keep an eye on your portions without having to constantly measure everything.

Listening to your satiety cues is another way to limit and monitor your total portion sizes. Just because you serve yourself three ounces of meat with supper every night doesn't mean this will be the perfect portion for you forever. This is where listening to your body is important. For example, on a day where you don't leave the house, two ounces of meat will likely be enough to satisfy your hunger. But on a day where you're helping a friend move in the morning, and doing yard work all afternoon, you may need three and a half ounces to feel satisfied.

Standard portion sizes are a good initial guide. Fine-tuning these portions based on your hunger level is the second step.

NOTE: If you're not satisfied on suggested WLS sized portions of food on a regular basis, you should meet with your WLS dietitian. This is often a sign that your meals and snacks are unbalanced, you're likely eating and drinking at the same time, and/or that you're not eating often enough. It's unlikely that you've re-stretched your stomach (a common fear of patients) especially in the first year after surgery.

Is it normal that I can't eat more than a ½ cup of food at a time?

This is a difficult question to answer.

It might be normal, just as much as it might mean something's wrong. If it's only been a few weeks since you had surgery, then it's absolutely normal that you can't eat more than a ½ cup of food. Everyone advances differently. Some patients will be able to eat one cup of food five to six weeks after surgery, but it takes most patients anywhere from two to six months after surgery to eat one cup of food comfortably. Some patients never get there even after a few years!

It's important to eat your food slowly, but to stop eating after 30 minutes. If you can't eat ½ cup of food in 30 minutes, and you're three to six months out, we strongly suggest that you contact your WLS team.

Your WLS team will ask you questions and may send you for testing to see why you're having difficulty. They may find an issue or they might just confirm that everything is normal. Either way, it's important that your team is aware so they can make sure everything is fine.

CHAPTER 13:

Eating Out

Three things I should NEVER leave home without

1. Water bottle

It's important to hydrate throughout the day, not just when you're at home or at work. Purchase a smaller-sized reusable water bottle (i.e. 500 mL) that's lighter to transport. Be sure not to leave it in the car, as this defeats the purpose of bringing it with you.

2. Emergency snack

Snacks that don't need refrigeration are ideal to keep in your purse or pockets. Keeping your energy up between meals by having snacks is the key to avoiding crashing and/or overeating later in the day.

Examples of good snacks include:

- ¼ cup nuts or seeds and some dried fruit;
- 2 tbsp peanut butter and some crackers;
- A soy milk tetra-pack;
- Protein bars;
- Protein drinks.

3. Plans for your next meal

Maintaining a regular eating schedule is super important no matter what your plans are for the day. Being too busy is not an excuse! Planning and being organized is truly the key to success after WLS.

Questions to ask yourself include:

- Will you be back home in time for your next meal?
- Should you pack a meal?
- Do your afternoon plans with friends include supper too?
- Do you plan to eat out? If so, where?

It'll take time, but these habits will soon become part of your daily routine. In the beginning, maintaining this checklist will require effort, but with time, it'll become intuitive.

What do I eat when I'm out of the house and stuck eating fast food?

If you're eating at a restaurant for *convenience*—meaning you weren't planning on eating out—you should choose a healthier option. This is bound to happen occasionally, whether it's because you didn't have time to pack your lunch or you forgot to do groceries last night. You don't want to reward your lack of planning and organization with a high calorie fast food meal!

Here are some tips for picking out the healthier options at the average fast food restaurant:

Sandwiches and wraps

Choose a sandwich on toasted bread. If it's a large sandwich, remove the top piece of bread. Great options include: chicken salad, egg salad, tuna salad, and deli meats. Wraps are also a great option. Opt for baked chicken rather than crispy chicken whenever possible.

Breakfast egg sandwiches

Choose a breakfast wrap or a toasted English muffin sandwich and skip the bacon and sausage.

Salads

Almost all restaurants have a green salad with chicken. Again, opt for grilled chicken instead of crispy chicken whenever possible. Other high protein options include taco salads, chickpea salads, and bean salads.

Chili

Whether you choose the vegetarian or meat version, chili packs a lot of protein. They're also easy to digest, making them the perfect option if you've only recently transitioned to solid food.

Sushi

You likely won't be able to tolerate your favourite sushi rolls because of the rice, but there are several other equally satisfying options on most Asian-style menus you should consider:

- Indulge in an order of tartar or sashimi, as these rice-less options are easier to digest;
- Don't be afraid to ask if your favourite sushi rolls can be made with a cucumber wrap instead of the traditional seaweed wrap (this is often a 'low carbohydrate' option on sushi menus);
- Order a side of edamame beans, which are both a good source of protein and fibre;

- Try a protein rich Asian soup which often has eggs, tofu, chicken, and/or shrimp. Leave the broth behind;
- Seared salmon or tuna over salad and a flavourful dressing.

Some other tips to remember:

- Skip the combo option even if it's cheaper.
- Don't order a drink. You'll be less tempted to drink and eat at the same time if you don't have a beverage staring you down during your meal.
- Eat in the restaurant instead of in the car. If you're driving and eating, food is more likely to block. You can't be mindful if you're multitasking!
- Choose foods described as: grilled, baked, sautéed, broiled, steamed, boiled, etc., as much as possible. These cooking methods are lower in calories.
- Many corner stores and gas stations now have 'grab and go' options in their fridges such as sandwiches, salads, protein shakes, yogurt parfaits, etc. Next time you get gas, make a note of three appropriate meal options you could choose if you were in a pinch.

CHAPTER 14:
Cooking, Not Cooking, & Meal Prep

What can I do when I don't feel like cooking supper?

The reality is, that no matter how much you enjoy cooking or how organized you are, there will be nights when you don't feel like cooking. For this reason, we want you to have some solid backup options.

Don't be afraid of canned food

Yes, canned foods are typically higher in salt, but they still make a healthier option in comparison to skipping a meal or eating fast food. Examples of items to choose include: canned chili, canned beans in tomato sauce, canned oysters or sardines with crackers, canned tuna with some mayo on toast, can of mixed beans with salad dressing and chopped vegetables, etc.

Pre-cooked BBQ chicken

Every large grocery store has them. The chicken is super versatile and leftovers make great lunches. You can add slices of chicken onto a salad, serve with rice and chopped veggies, add mayo or mustard and make a sandwich or wrap, or mix in with some pasta and sauce.

Frozen meals

Yes, frozen meals are typically higher in salt and fat than home-cooked meals, but we like that they're portion-controlled and, again, compared to skipping a meal or opting for fast food, they're still the healthier option.

Breakfast for supper

There's nothing wrong with choosing a lower prep breakfast option for supper. Examples include yogurt and fruit, toast and peanut butter, an omelette, one or two boiled eggs with toast, oatmeal made with milk, etc.

How do I choose a frozen meal?

When selecting a frozen meal, it's important to consider several factors: nutritional value, personal tastes, and your tolerance to certain foods. If you know that rice and pasta simply won't go down since having surgery, it's a better idea to select the frozen meals that don't use these foods as the main element.

When considering nutritional value you will need to look at the nutrition facts table and opt for meals with:

Nutrition Facts
Valeur nutritive
Per 1 frozen meal / Pour 1 repas surgelé ☆

Amount Teneur	% Daily Value % valeur quotidienne
Calories / Calories 300 - 350 ☆	
Fat / Lipides	%
Saturated / saturés + Trans / trans	%
Cholesterol / Cholestérol	
Sodium / Sodium 400 mg max ☆	%
Carbohydrate / Glucides	
Fibre / Fibres	
Sugars / Sucres	
Protein / Protéines min 15 g ☆	
Vitamin A / Vitamine A	%
Vitamin C / Vitamine C	%
Calcium / Calcium	%
Iron / Fer	%

- A maximum of 300-350 calories per portion (i.e. the whole frozen meal);
- A minimum of 15 g of protein per portion (most of the pasta-based frozen meals will not contain enough protein);
- 400 mg of sodium (salt) or less. It's very difficult to find a frozen meal that's low in salt, but try your best.

If there are frozen dinners that contain an added packet of sweet sauce to add after warming, use this minimally as they usually contain a lot of extra sugar, salt, and fat. So add just enough to suit your taste.

What do I do for lunch if I have a difficulty preparing it ahead of time?

Bringing a homemade lunch to work will not only save you money, but it'll also save you from extra fat and salt, and reduce your risk of unwanted tolerance issues in front of your colleagues. If you're notorious at the office for not bringing a lunch to work, consider some of the following options.

Use leftovers

Pack leftovers directly into your lunch container immediately after supper for the following day. The leftovers need to be put away regardless, so you might as well divide them up into meal-sized portions now, rather than doing it in the morning as you're running out the door.

Frozen meal alternatives

Homemade food is always best, but convenient frozen meals are an okay option every once in awhile, especially if you're debating eating out or skipping lunch instead. A couple of frozen meals can be left in the freezer at work at the beginning of every month for days where you forget to pack a lunch or are too busy to make something the night before. Ideally, bring some pre-cut veggies or a fruit to have on the side too.

Ready-to-eat options

How close is the nearest grocery store from your work? Do you drive by one on your morning commute?

Most grocery stores have a ready-to-eat food section near the deli. This is divided up into the fried food section (fried chicken, chicken wings, and French fries), the home-cooked meal section (shepherd's pie, meatballs in tomato sauce with rice, and roasted chicken), the salad bar (lettuce, vegetables, tuna, boiled eggs, roasted chicken), and the chilled grab-and-go section (prepared lentil and quinoa salads, egg salad wraps, cheese/hummus/cracker/vegetable combos). Avoid fried foods and choose something from one of the other three sections.

Preparing homemade meals and snacks is always preferred, but the reality is that most people lead busy lives. Knowing what your options are outside of the fast food world is important after WLS.

CHAPTER 15:

Self-monitoring

Why use a food journal?

No one likes keeping a food journal. We know. It's tedious, time-consuming, and can be a bit of a hassle. But keeping track of your food choices, portions, and timing of your meals and snacks for several days in a row can provide you with incredibly valuable information. It provides a snapshot of where you're at in terms of your eating habits. It provides us (your WLS dietitians) with the opportunity to review, provide feedback, reflect, question, and troubleshoot, to further tweak and improve your current eating habits.

Here's another way to think about it: how would you know how much money you have in your bank account if the bank didn't send you monthly statements? How would you know how much gas you have in your car if there wasn't a gas gauge? What about the battery level on your cell phone? How would a library know where their books are if they didn't keep tabs on them?

We lead busy lives and our minds can't keep track of everything we do or be 100% self-aware at all times. It's not humanly possible.

We've seen many patients write food journals by listing the food they eat on a blank piece of paper like this:

- Sandwich;
- Banana;

- Yogurt.

Unfortunately, this list is extremely incomplete. There are so many questions that are left unanswered, including:

- What was in the sandwich (i.e. did it have a source of protein?)?
- Was it a 6" sub, 12" sub, one or two slices of bread?
- Was it on white bread or whole grain bread?
- Was it homemade or purchased?
- Did you finish all of it?
- How long did it take you to eat it?
- What time was it when you ate it?
- When was the last time you ate?
- Did you feel hungry when you decided to eat it?
- Did you feel satisfied, comfortable, or full when you were done eating?
- How long after the sandwich did you eat again?
- Where did you eat it?
- Did you drink anything with the sandwich?
- If you drank something, what was it?

And we haven't even asked questions about the banana and yogurt yet!

The answers to all of these questions should ideally be included in a food journal. Why? Because they help answer the most important questions related to what you ate, how much you ate, why you ate it, why you had certain tolerance issues, how satisfied you were, etc.

In our opinion, the main purpose of food journals isn't to count calories—which is what food apps typically focus on and what many patients obsess over—but to be used as a tool in order to better understand your eating habits. We basically want to zero in on what's working for you and what's not working for you as quickly as possible. A detailed food journal allows us to do this.

We've had many patients who've tracked everything they ate for three days and of the ones who take it seriously, they always learn something about themselves. How can you change a habit if you don't recognize it in the first place? You need to be aware of your habits and take the time to reflect on them. Basic food journaling can help with this.

Just like anything else in life, the more effort you put in, the more you'll get out of the experience.

Why does my dietitian ask me to keep a food journal?

Pharmacists can only help you if you bring them a prescription from a doctor. Mortgage companies can only help you if you bring a summary of your finances. And teachers can only help you if you've completed yesterday's homework. Similarly, dietitians can only begin to help you if you bring a complete and *thoughtful*, food journal. It's the basis of our conversation and provides us with the information needed to help with your concerns.

Remember that we are not asking you to food journal every day for the rest of your life. That would be ridiculously cruel! We are simply asking for 3 days of journals at each appointment.

How often should I weigh myself?

In our opinion, weighing yourself one to two times per week is more than enough. After WLS we see many of our patients weighing themselves daily, and even up to several times a day. This habit can do more harm than good. You won't see the pounds melt away between noon and dinner. However, you *will* see a change over a one week period. Your body doesn't gain or lose weight over a 24-hour period. Our metabolism runs continuously at different rates throughout the day and averages out over a three to four day period. Any minor fluctuations that you see on the scale (i.e. up or down 1-4 lbs) over the course of the day shouldn't be taken seriously.

CHAPTER 16:
Physical Activity

If I eat really healthy do I still need to exercise?

If we told you that we had the answer to how you could prevent weight regain, improve your heart health, diabetes, and high blood pressure, improve your mood, boost your self-esteem, increase your energy, improve your sleep, and much much more, would you want in?

Of course you would!

It turns out exercise does all of this!

So, if you eat really healthy, do you still need to exercise? If you're still not answering yes, we suggest you re-read the paragraph above.

Should I have a snack before or after I exercise?

This entirely depends on how you feel. We definitely suggest a snack before and after, but read on for details.

If you feel hungry while exercising, or feel that you get tired within the first few minutes of exercising and can't push yourself to finish your workout, then you probably need a snack before exercising. Plan to have a snack within two hours before working out. This can be one to two tablespoons of peanut butter on a slice of whole wheat bread, or it can be ½ cup of a fibre cereal with milk (i.e. a carbohydrate and protein snack, low in fat, so it's easy to digest). If you didn't have time to eat your snack two hours before exercising, but feel tired early into exercising, you should have a carbohydrate snack, such as a fruit (one fruit the size of your fist, or ½ cup of fruit salad), within the hour before working out. This will give you the sugar boost that your body needs to reduce the fatigue and allow you to push yourself during your workout.

It's important to take advantage of the state your body's in after exercising, which is the anabolic state. This means that your body is in its replenishing mode to stock up on the sugar you burned off while exercising. Your body stores sugar in your liver and in your muscles. This is important in controlling your blood sugar during the periods that you're not eating (like during the night). Your liver helps control your blood sugar by releasing small amounts of sugar when your levels drop overnight. After exercising, your body also wants to repair the muscles that you used, particularly during resistance activities like weight training or high resistance biking. For these reasons, you should have a snack after working out that includes some carbohydrates and some protein.

Most research will agree that in order to take advantage of this muscle repair window, it is best to have protein within 30 to 60 minutes of exercising. This is when your body will benefit most from protein to repair your muscles. If you aren't eating a meal within an hour of exercising, pack a healthy snack to eat after the gym (e.g. one cup of milk, 100 g of flavoured Greek yogurt, or one and a half ounces of cheese with two large crackers or four small crackers).

NOTE: These suggestions are for mild to moderate activity for up to one and a half hours. If you're engaging in intense physical activity (e.g.

training for a marathon or fitness competition) then you should consult your WLS dietitian or a sports dietitian. Additionally, sports gels and energy chews may cause dumping in gastric bypass patients. Speak with your dietitian to learn more about appropriate mid-workout snacks for long high-intensity workouts, races, or competitions.

Hydration

Don't forget to sip on water throughout your workout. When you're exercising you want to be able to give it your all, in order to get the health benefits from cardiovascular and weight resistance exercises. The more you sweat and the heavier you breathe while exercising, the more water you're losing from your body. If you don't replace the water that you're losing, you can become dehydrated which can lead to feeling increasingly tired early into your workout.

Depending on the intensity of your exercise, sip on water every 15 to 20 minutes. Water alone is enough for a 60 minute workout. Sports drinks with electrolytes are not usually needed unless you're intensely active and sweating for more than an hour at a time. If you weigh yourself before and after exercise on the same scale, you'll see that you may have lost a very small amount of weight. This shows you the amount of water that you lost while exercising. If you lose more than 2% of your body weight after exercising, you aren't drinking enough during your workout.

What can I do for exercise aside from going to the gym?

If gyms simply aren't your thing or your finances are tight, there are many other things you can do to exercise regularly that don't involve going to a gym or fitness club.

Check out YouTube
Find a YouTube exercise channel that you like and subscribe to their page to receive a notice when a new video is posted. YouTube has exercise videos for aerobics, zumba, yoga, pilates, weight training, you name it! There are even videos for patients who may need extra support due to bad knees or back pain.

Go for a walk
Walking is a great activity, but we suggest that you invest in a pedometer to count your steps. Exercise is best when you can track your progress and counting your steps is a great, simple, and low cost way of doing so. Speed walking or choosing roads with a bit of an incline are good ways to increase the intensity.

You can also join a walking group in your area, or create one on a social media support group. Connect with other patients who have had WLS surgery who live close by and start a club. Plus, if you have great outdoor walking or hiking trails nearby, you can walk them for free or for a low cost annual membership.

Be thrifty
Elastic resistance bands can be found for a low cost at big box stores. We've even seen exercise equipment at both discount and dollar stores!

If you have a smartphone, there are countless free apps you can download to help you increase your activity during the day. Try one out each day until you find one you like.

What does your community offer for free? Do your research. Some fitness classes are by donation and many YMCAs offer free swim hours for locals.

Try taking up badminton in your yard, walking the dog, gardening, or pushing your children or grandkids on a swing. These are great ways to start feeling good about moving your body again without overdoing it to start.

The important thing is to find something you like. Don't feel bad about getting bored of an activity! Just pick up another one until you find something that makes you happy. Keep it interesting and don't be afraid to try new types of activities.

The bottom line: If you don't enjoy the activity, it's not going to last long!

CHAPTER 17:
Vitamins & Mineral Supplements

If I eat well, why do I need to take daily vitamins?

Even if you have three balanced meals and two to three balanced snacks every day after WLS, you're still almost guaranteed to develop multiple vitamin and mineral deficiencies if you're not taking daily vitamins. There are two main reasons for this.

First of all, and most obviously, you're no longer able to consume large enough amounts of foods to meet your micronutrient (i.e. vitamin and mineral) needs.

Secondly, your body now absorbs and processes foods differently. For example, if you had a malabsorptive weight loss surgery (e.g. gastric bypass or duodenal switch), in addition to eating smaller portions of foods, you're also not absorbing 100% of the nutrients in the foods that you're eating. Interestingly, even in the non-malabsorptive procedures (e.g. sleeve gastrectomy and band) we see changes in nutrient processing. For example, you may no longer have enough stomach acid in your small stomach to efficiently absorb the natural calcium found in dairy products, which is why you've been prescribed a special type of calcium, calcium *citrate*, that doesn't require stomach acid to be absorbed.

The signs and symptoms of vitamin and mineral deficiencies can be mild to severe. Some take only weeks to occur, while others take years to develop. While many deficiencies are reversible (e.g. anemia, or low iron), several micronutrient deficiencies are irreversible (e.g. osteoporosis, or bone decay due to inadequate calcium and vitamin D, and neurological damage due to inadequate B vitamins).

Moral of the story? Take your vitamins!

How can a WLS dietitian be of assistance with vitamins and deficiencies?

Your WLS dietitian can quickly identify if you have any severe micronutrient deficiencies with a simple visual exam of your scalp, face and hands. They can also identify mild to moderate deficiencies based on your list of symptoms. Your WLS team will then recommend blood tests be done to confirm any suspicions. Your surgeon or family doctor can then prescribe the necessary vitamins.

There are so many formats and brands of vitamins on the market. If you're not taking your vitamins because you don't like the taste of them, or you feel like you're taking ten pills a day, let your WLS dietitian know! Don't use this as an excuse to stop taking them. Your dietitian will work with you to find a vitamin format that fits your lifestyle (e.g. chewable, liquid, dissolves under the tongue, pill), a schedule that works for you, and possibly reduce the number of vitamins you take in a day (i.e. by introducing you to WLS specific brands of vitamins).

If your family doctor doesn't know what blood tests they should be ordering for you, your WLS dietitian will be more than happy to provide a list of what should be tested and how often your blood should be screened. Depending on what type of weight loss surgery you've had, blood tests should be done every three to six months in the first year after surgery and every six to 12 months annually in the years after WLS.

How often do I need to have blood tests?

Your WLS team will tell you how often you should have blood tests done. It's most likely that you'll have a blood test after your surgery, while you're still in the hospital. Following this, your next blood test will be in three to six months and continue every three to six months until your first year after surgery, depending on the type of surgery you had. If your blood tests are looking great at one year after surgery, this is a good sign and means that you managed to get through the first risky year after WLS without having developed a deficiency!

But this doesn't mean that blood tests are no longer needed. You'll need to do blood tests to check for nutrient deficiencies for the rest of your life. As you get older, your body needs more of some nutrients and less of others as your body changes. Some deficiencies also take a longer time to develop. For this reason, you may still develop deficiencies over time, even five to ten years after surgery. We've seen many patients who stopped doing their blood tests because they felt fine only to find out years later that they have multiple severe deficiencies. Feeling good doesn't mean everything is good. And there's a reason why.

Before feeling tired, lethargic, weak, or sick, because of a nutrient deficiency, your body goes through the following stages:

- You're not getting enough of a nutrient from your diet and your vitamins;
- Your body doesn't have enough of the nutrient stored;
- You begin to have low levels of the nutrient in your body;

- Your organs begin to have trouble working properly;
- You begin feeling unwell and develop symptoms of deficiencies.

Feeling unwell is the *last* step in this process.

These steps can take only a few weeks for some nutrients, and up to several months for others. When you begin to feel unwell, your body has already been through weeks—or months—of missing an important nutrient. Blood tests can catch these deficiencies at a much earlier stage.

For example, say you stopped taking your iron pill. You wouldn't feel an anemia, or an iron deficiency, developing. Gradually, over time, you'll begin to get tired and you might figure it's just your busy lifestyle. You'll begin to feel worse and wonder if you're just not getting enough sleep. Then you'll become increasingly lethargic and notice your hair has lost its shine and is getting brittle. Lastly, you'll notice that you can hardly get through your morning routine without having to sit down and take a break. You'll go to your doctor who will order blood tests. The blood tests will come back diagnosing you with anemia. Luckily, you'll restart your iron supplement which will reverse this condition, although it'll take about three months until you feel like yourself again. However, some deficiencies aren't reversible which can leave you unwell permanently.

The bottom line: Have your blood tests done regularly as suggested by your WLS team. You'll eventually only have one blood test per year, but this will only be the case at two years after WLS or until your blood tests routinely come back normal. If you no longer see your WLS team, or live too far from your WLS centre, make sure that your family doctor is testing you for WLS-related deficiencies. The routine blood tests that your family doctor performs aren't the same ones that your WLS team orders. We look at so much more. Ask your family doctor if he/she is looking for all the nutrients necessary for WLS. They can receive this information from the WLS clinic where you had your surgery.

CHAPTER 18:
Emotional Changes & Support

Emotional changes

Life after WLS is filled with changes. Obviously there are changes to your lifestyle and eating habits, but what many patients aren't able to anticipate before surgery is that WLS touches on all aspects of your life. Here's a short list of the, at times, underappreciated changes:

- Changes in your relationships (romantic, familial and friend);
- Excess skin;
- Eating at restaurants/socially;
- Identifying as a lower weight person;
- Judgement from others for 'taking the easy way out' by having surgery (which, as this book shows, is 100% untrue);
- Giving up life-long habits;
- Coping with life-long maintenance of these new habits.

Many of our patients struggle with no longer being able to manage their stress with their favourite foods or alcohol. Some patients experience a return of old addictions (e.g. drugs, gambling, shopping, etc.) or new episodes of depression or social anxiety.

Everyone reacts differently. Everyone has different coping mechanisms.

It's important to seek help if you're not adjusting to life after surgery well. If you feel overwhelmed, more anxious than usual, alone, or depressed, please reach out to your WLS centre as soon as possible. If your WLS centre has long wait times for appointments, reach out to your family doctor or a local psychologist.

If you're contemplating hurting yourself, we urge you to call emergency services.

Life after surgery affects everyone differently, but you don't have to suffer alone.

The importance of support

It's important to develop a good support system after surgery. Your new habits will touch on all aspects of your life. You're going to hit some lows and rough patches, but this is normal. Lifestyle changes and developing a new relationship with food is *hard*. For this reason, it's a good idea, in preparation for WLS, to start building a community of support.

Support comes in many different forms:

- Your WLS team (i.e. dietitian, nurse, psychologist, surgeon);
- Family;
- Close friends;
- Work colleagues (this of course is a personal choice);
- Your family doctor;

- In-person support groups (ask your WLS team for details on local groups);
- Online support groups (like social media groups, online forums, blogs, recipe sites, etc.);
- WLS apps (these will help support your new dietary changes);
- WLS podcasts;
- New technology (like step-counters).

Is it possible to develop disordered eating habits after WLS?

Yes. It's definitely possible to develop disordered or obsessive eating habits after surgery. Many of our patients, especially those who track everything in food diary apps, become too focused on the numbers and forget to look at the big picture (like enjoying wholesome, nourishing, flavourful foods). These patients want to know targets, limits, and ranges for their daily calories, carbohydrates, fat and sugar, down to the decimal!

It's important to keep in mind that while weight management comes down to the numbers, calculating everything you eat, every day, for the rest of your life isn't realistic nor normal behaviour. It's more sustainable to apply the concepts discussed in this book that encourage a better relationship with food than to count your calories daily.

In our experience, disordered eating most commonly starts when our patients are transitioning onto solid foods after surgery. Re-introducing trigger foods such as bread, pasta, and sweets can be really scary. Patients often don't know how to incorporate these types of foods in moderation, or they don't trust themselves not to overeat, so they overcompensate by deciding to completely avoid them.

All foods fit after surgery. Finding a 'new normal' and learning to trust and respect your body and new stomach takes time. If you feel like you're having a hard time introducing trigger foods in moderation, or if you feel anxious around your food diary app, contact a dietitian who specializes in working with WLS patients.

A Final Word from the Authors

Our wish for you, is that:

- You find moderation and balance with all foods;
- You don't lose the pleasure in eating;
- You embrace your journey;
- You find your best weight and celebrate it;
- You learn to listen for and trust your body's cues;
- You develop new habits that will last a lifetime;
- You let go of diet language and see right through the latest weight loss fad;
- You won't be afraid to seek help when you feel alone;
- You focus on the positive changes in your quality of life that WLS has brought you;
- You be kind to your fellow WLS patients;
- You find peace within.

Whether you're simply contemplating the idea of surgery, have your surgery booked, or have already undergone surgery, we hope this book serves as a useful tool in your journey.

If you've benefited from this book, we'd love to hear from you! Messages from beautiful people like *you* are why we're so passionate about what we do.

You can email us at: bariatricsurgerynutrition@gmail.com.

If you're interested in working one-on-one with us, joining one of our online small group workshops, or need meal plan support, check out our website: www.bariatricsurgerynutrition.com.

On our website you can also sign up for our free newsletter. By signing up, you'll receive monthly blog posts and WLS tips right to your inbox. You'll also be the first to know about our newest WLS services and products.

And lastly, show us some love by liking our Facebook page: Bariatric Surgery Nutrition. Subscribing to our page is the easiest way to stay up to date with us. We regularly post tips, recipes, recommended content (e.g. podcasts, books, movies, etc.) and much, much more!

Made in the USA
Columbia, SC
03 August 2021

42924572R00080